Scale Down—Live It Up
Wellness Workbook

Scale Down—Live It Up
Wellness Workbook

Danna Demetre

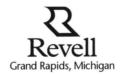

Revell

Grand Rapids, Michigan

Published by Fleming H. Revell
a division of Baker Publishing Group
P.O. Box 6287, Grand Rapids, MI 49516-6287
www.revellbooks.com

Printed in the United States of America

ISBN 0-8007-3127-1

Unless otherwise indicated, Scripture is taken from the New American Standard Bible®, Copyright © 1960, 1962, 1963, 1968, 1971, 1972, 1973, 1975, 1977, 1995 by The Lockman Foundation. Used by permission.

Scripture marked NIV is taken from the HOLY BIBLE, NEW INTERNATIONAL VERSION®. NIV®. Copyright © 1973, 1978, 1984 by International Bible Society. Used by permission of Zondervan. All rights reserved.

This publication is designed to provide accurate and authoritative information in regard to the subject matter covered. Whenever starting a new fitness or exercise program, LifeStyle Dimensions recommends a medical checkup first from a competent physician.

The Personality Profile on pages 130–34 is used by permission of CLASServices Inc. If you would like to order the Personality Profile, please contact CLASServices at 3311 Candelaria NE Suite 1, Albuquerque, NM 87107, or call (800) 433-6633 or use the website www.classervices.com.

Contents

Introduction

In This Section:

Perhaps you remember a television commercial in which a young delivery service employee is instructed to transport a package as quickly as possible to "Fargo." He accepts the assignment with great enthusiasm and jumps into his car for a nonstop trip across the country, reaching Fargo, North Dakota, in record time. As he picks up the package to double-check the address, he notices something very important. The package reads, "John Fargo, Suite 300." Oops. The package was supposed to be delivered to a man named Fargo in the same building! It pays to pay attention to details.

Got a Plan?

Having the right information before starting on any journey is really important. I believe the *Scale Down—Live It Up* program and workbook will give you the best road map to reach your ultimate destination: a leaner, healthier body and a more balanced soul and spirit. This workbook is designed to augment the *Scale Down* book and the six-part CD or DVD program. You certainly can use the workbook with the book alone, but you will have much greater success if you use all the tools available.

Watching or listening to the *Scale Down—Live It Up* program more than once during your eight-week journey will greatly enhance your ability to internalize and implement all that you are learning. You may choose to move at a faster or slower pace than I have designed; that's up to you! You need to realize that you are not beginning an "eight-week program." Rather, this workbook will help you understand and implement the principles necessary to achieve a truly victorious lifestyle for a lifetime.

Workbook Schedule

You will note that this workbook is designed for you to watch or listen to one session from the *Scale Down—Live It Up* program in each of the first six weeks. In the seventh week, you will dig a little deeper into the subject of calorie control, nutritious eating, and sharing healthy recipes. Week eight is dedicated to the "click factor"—that is, helping you discover your unique "motivating factors" and how to customize your self-talk to renew your mind in key areas. Finally, week nine, "A Personality-Powered Lifestyle," is an optional session you can do in a group or on your own. It will help you understand some of the ways your temperament may influence how you make lasting lifestyle change.

Pace Yourself

Whether you are going through the program as a self-study or in a group, feel free to move ahead at your own pace. If you have the time, getting the whole picture in the first couple weeks and then going back through more slowly can be very helpful for those who want to get a jump start on their new lifestyle. Conversely, if the pace is too fast, simply slow down and process the information and assignments as you can. Too often, when people get overwhelmed, they simply quit or drop out. Don't do that! Commit yourself to the process, and over time you will find small victories adding up to bigger victories that will reflect themselves in your body in tangible ways.

This journey toward lifestyle victory has many aspects that go far beyond simply changing your eating and exercise habits. Don't get overwhelmed. Remind yourself that this is a journey that will take time. Once you have the "big picture," go back to your specific areas of weakness and concentrate on those. Just as we don't read the Bible once and put it down never to pick it up again, you will need to go back and reread and review some chapters.

The Power of Multiple Mediums

Research reveals that using multiple mediums (written, auditory, and visual) can improve learning dramatically. The *Scale Down—Live It Up* DVD and CD programs will enhance your ability to learn and implement the principles taught in my book. If you are watching the DVDs in a group setting, I highly recommend getting your own copy of the program in CD form. Listen to it while exercising, driving, or doing mundane tasks. The more often you input new information, the more easily you will be able to make it real in your own life. In addition, try to teach someone else the most important principles you learn in each session. The act of teaching will help you internalize the concepts.

Helpful Weight Loss Tools

In the course of this program, you will read about and hear me refer to several weight loss tools that have been of great help to thousands of my clients over the last decade. Should you want to learn more about resources such as my biblically grounded *Healthy Self-Talk* CD or the Caltrac activity monitor, visit my website at www.dannademetre.com.

Partner Up for Greater Success

We can't deny that teaming up with one other person or more has tremendous benefit. Exchange phone numbers and email addresses and stay in touch once a week. You can even meet at the gym, take a walk together, or enjoy a healthy lunch together. Pray for each other. Share your frustrations and successes. If you are not in a group program, I encourage you to find a friend who will join you and travel this lifestyle journey together. You could even begin a small group of your own.

Group Programs

If you do get your own group together, be sure to order a *Scale Down— Live It Up Leader's Guide*. It will give you helpful direction on how to lead a group effectively. I recommend that you view one DVD per week in the first six weeks of your group program. Use this workbook to dig deeper into the subject covered, complete personal evaluations, and design a lifestyle "recipe" in each key area. You will also find key Scriptures and personal reflection or discussion questions at the end of each session. The studies can be done on your own or as part of a group, using the questions as topics for group discussion.

Making the Most of Scale Down

Don't get overwhelmed as you begin to dig in to these materials. Just remember that small steps, taken consistently, add up in a big way over time. Your first small step is to take one week at a time and try to complete the simple assignments.

Weekly Format

The workbook follows a consistent format each week which includes the following elements:

1. Follow-along Outline

This section allows you to take notes and fill in some blanks as you watch or listen to the *Scale Down—Live It Up* programs in the first six weeks.

2. Personal Reflection

After each week's teaching, this section allows you to ask yourself some specific questions related to that week's topics. This can be done either individually or as part of a group discussion. Do be sure to jot down your initial thoughts and ideas and reflect on them later in the week.

3. Build a Strong Spiritual Foundation

This section digs into some Scripture related to the subjects. Again, you are asked to write your personal thoughts. If you are part of a group, this may be a good time to connect with two to four others and share on a more personal level. If you are doing the program alone, this section would be excellent for your devotions or quiet time once or twice during the week.

4. Nourish Your Spirit

You will notice that each week, I encourage you to focus on four specific spiritual disciplines. They are:

1. Pray as if it is the air you breathe
2. Nourish your soul and spirit with God's Word daily
3. Digest its truths through meditation
4. Practice the presence of God

You will also note that each week's emphasis in these areas differs depending upon the subject matter. So don't assume that you've already covered these issues when you see the same headings each week. Take the time to dig deep, invest in your spiritual growth, and surrender all your lifestyle challenges to God.

Obviously, this exercise needs to be done alone. Again, I recommend that you devote at least one day's devotional time to this exercise. Then try to bring these disciplines to mind throughout your week as you go about your daily activities. So much of your long-term change will depend upon your commitment to "setting your mind on things above" (see Col. 3:2).

5. Prayer for Each Week

For each week I have written a prayer specific to that week's focus. I hope you will use it as an example of how you can be praying as you release all your struggles to God and seek his supernatural intervention in your life.

6. Suggested Reading

Each week, you will also be encouraged to read the corresponding chapters in the *Scale Down* book. If you have already read the book, I recommend at least skimming the chapters once again to reinforce those concepts that are not included in the DVDs or CDs. Those of you who are not "readers," please do read the entire book. It includes many concepts and illustrations that simply could not be included in the *Scale Down—Live It Up* materials. You will miss some very important teaching if you choose not to read the book in its entirety.

Personal Evaluations

You will also notice that after each key area of teaching you will be instructed to take a personal evaluation. Those key areas are: (1) Perspective/Motivation, (2) Burning Fat, (3) Nutrition, and (4) Fitness. After taking the evaluation and computing your score, you find on the following pages a "menu" of healthy principles or actions and a "recipe" page where you can choose the top three priorities you want to focus on in this area of your life. You will find it helpful to transfer your "recipe" to an index card or into your day planner if you use one. That way you can refer to it occasionally during the week and remind yourself of your plan.

I also recommend retaking the evaluations periodically as you progress in your lifestyle journey. Use a different color ink each time. Take some time to review these evaluations and put your greatest attention on the area of your greatest weakness.

As you progress through each of the weekly assignments, please realize that you don't need to complete every single assignment. You may be strong in an area that you can simply skip. On the other hand, in some areas you may need more time. The eight-week guide is simply a way to systematically ingest and begin to apply many mental, physical, and spiritual principles to your life.

Logging for Success

Near the end of this workbook, you will find some helpful tools for logging your lifestyle progress. Some people find that they do better and are more motivated when they keep daily records. Others like to keep things very simple. That is why it is very important that you use tools and make changes that you can live with—changes that fit with your life and personality.

Initial Evaluation: Gaining Perspective

You are about to embark on a journey with *Scale Down*. The following questions will help you understand your personal desires and level of commitment from the outset.

1. What physical, mental, emotional, and spiritual changes do you hope to achieve?

2. Why is this important to you?

3. For whom do you want to make these changes or improvements?

4. How do you think they will change your life?

5. What will it cost you (in time, energy, money, etc.)?

6. Are you willing to pay that price?

7. Do you believe you can do this with God's help?

Okay, now it's time to get started with the program. I recommend that you spend a few minutes every day reading your *Scale Down* book and reflecting on the key spiritual perspectives in that section. I've heard it said that "we make time for that which is most important to us." If this is true and your body and health are important to you, please make the time. It will be well worth it.

Week One:
The Body Battle

In This Section:

The Three Keys to Permanent Weight Loss
Seven Small Steps to Permanent Change

Follow-along Outline

View or listen to session one as you fill in the blanks in this outline and jot down your own notes or thoughts in the margins. Then complete the workbook assignments for this week at the end of this section individually or with your group.

Knowing what to do is easy. Getting yourself to do it . . . now that's the challenge!

Scale Down *Overview*

- Understanding the balance of body, soul, and spirit
- Realizing that "you are what you think"
- Discovering the power of your true identity
- Accessing the weapons to fight the "battle of the flesh"

- Eating for high energy and health
- Burning fat to the max

The Three Keys to Permanent Weight Loss

The Lies

A supplement or pill will solve your problems.

You must "diet" to lose weight.

You can lose a pound a day!

The Truth

There are no quick fixes or magic bullets . . . it's up to _____!

It takes more time to _____weight than _____ weight.

You have to lose weight the _____ way you plan to keep it off.

To lose weight permanently, you have to take it off the same way you plan to keep it off. The only realistic way is through a lifestyle change. Ask yourself this question: "Can I eat and exercise this way most days for _____?"

If the answer is no, you've just gone on another diet!

Key #1: The Body

Present your bodies as a living and holy sacrifice, acceptable to God, which is your spiritual service of worship.

Romans 12:1

1. The bottom line to losing excess fat is simply _____ in versus _____ out!

2. FACT: The average person gains 25 pounds between the ages of 30 and 50 years old. Question: How many extra calories must be consumed each day for this to happen?
   A. 5 to 10   B. 50 to 100   C. 250 to 300

3. The average American woman burns _____ calories per day:
   A. 1,000–1,200   B. 1,300–1,500   C. 1,600–1,700

4. If I burn 100 calories more than I eat each day, it will take me _____ days to burn off one pound of fat.

THE 100 CALORIE RULE:

For every 100 calories "extra" you burn each day, you will lose about ten pounds of fat off your body each YEAR.

THE 500 CALORIE RULE:

For every 500 calories "extra" you burn each day, you will lose about one pound of fat off your body each WEEK or 52 pounds each YEAR.

We build a completely new body every _____ years.

Therefore, I must remember each and every day that I _____ what I _____!

Key #2: The Soul

Do not be conformed to this world, but be transformed by the renewing of your mind.

Romans 12:2

1. Your mind is the _____ of your _____.

2. To change your habits or behavior, you must first change your

   _____.

3. In the human brain, the most _____ thought wins.

4. To change your mind, you must _____ and _____ old negative programs.

5. Before you can change unhealthy thinking, you must identify the _____ you believe and replace them with _____.

GET A NEW ATTITUDE

- The "All or Nothing" Attitude
- The "Quit Before You Start" Attitude
- The "I Don't Have Time" Attitude
- Get a _____ Attitude!

Key #3: The Spirit

Whether, then, you eat or drink or whatever you do, do all to the glory of God.

1 Corinthians 10:31

1. _____ your goals and desires for your body, mind, and spirit to God.
2. He who walks by the Spirit will not fulfill the desires of the _____.
3. Pray for enough _____ for the moment.
4. Ask yourself this question: Does this attitude, behavior, eating plan, or lifestyle _____ God?

"God will not give us good habits; He will not give us character; He will not make us walk aright. We have to do that for ourselves. Beware of the tendency of asking the way when you know it perfectly well."

Oswald Chambers

5. _____ as if it is the air you breathe.
6. _____ your spirit with God's Word daily.

Seven Small Steps to Permanent Change

1. Evaluate your lifestyle in four key areas:

   (a) _____

(b) _____

(c) _____

(d) _____

2. Grow in knowledge about _____ and _____.

3. Find ways to eat fewer _____ each day.

4. Burn more calories by moving _____ each day.

5. Measure your success by changes in your attitude and behavior, not the _____.

6. Renew your mind with _____.

7. Do the right things for the right reasons . . . and _____ the results!

Small steps, taken consistently, add up in a BIG way over time!

Review these checkpoints toward a victorious lifestyle daily:

Consider putting these checkpoints on an index card or somewhere in your daily planner where you can review them daily to remind you of the healthy, positive perspectives that will help you reach your long-term lifestyle goals.

☐ I am finding creative ways to eat fewer calories every day.

☐ I am finding simple ways to burn more calories every day.

☐ I am learning to eat for maximum energy and health.

☐ I am making purposeful activity or exercise a regular habit.

☐ I am identifying and changing my unhealthy beliefs and attitudes.

☐ I am building a foundation of truth from God's Word in order to live victoriously.

☐ I am becoming transformed by the renewing of my mind.

☐ I am learning to see myself and my goals through God's eyes.

Personal Reflection

Answer the following questions on your own or with your group:

1. Identify the most damaging "lie" you believe that is sabotaging your lifestyle success and write it here:

2. What new attitude is the single most important one for you to work on during your *Scale Down* journey? Write it here:

3. Decide on three ways to eat fewer calories this week and write them below:

    (a) _____

    (b) _____

    (c) _____

4. Determine three ways to burn more calories this week and write them below:

    (a) _____

    (b) _____

    (c) _____

Build a Strong Spiritual Foundation

Meditate on this Scripture and answer the corresponding questions:

Offer your bodies as living sacrifices, holy and pleasing to God, this is your spiritual act of worship.

Romans 12:1

1. Why is it so difficult to present our bodies as living sacrifices?

2. How can you begin to truly see your body as a means of worshiping God?

3. Do you think this awareness will help you in changing your lifestyle?

Nourish Your Spirit

Life-changing spiritual victory requires daily nourishment. Nourish your spirit daily in four ways:

1. Pray as if it is the air you breathe.

Pray the prayer below this week, surrendering every dimension of your life to the Lord. Add your own thoughts and words each day and give God your entire life—body, soul, and spirit.

2. Nourish your soul and spirit with God's Word daily.

Read and reread Romans 12:1 and ask God to show you how this Scripture relates to you personally.

3. Digest its truths through meditation.

Imagine God's pleasure as you present your body as a living sacrifice. See him delighting as you make sacrifices in your lifestyle because you know he is pleased when you take good care of yourself and invest in your long-term health and energy.

4. Practice the presence of God.

Remind yourself throughout the day that God is constantly with you and cares about all the details of your life. He loves you just the way you are but truly wants the very best for you as you walk and live in this physical world.

Prayer for Week One

Lord, I commit this journey to you. I pray that you will be glorified as I seek wisdom and strength to do "the right things for the right reasons." Thank you for the incredible body you have given me. I present it as a living sacrifice. Please help me to glorify you in it as I move out of bondage to my unhealthy thinking and habits. Show me where I'm believing lies. Help me to replace those lies with truth. In Jesus's name, Amen.

Suggested Reading for Week One

Read the following chapters and check off below:

☐ *Chapter 1: The Battle of the Body*

- "I hate my body! What about you?"
- Danna's personal story

☐ *Chapter 2: Getting Started*

- It's just four short pages. . . . You can do it!

☐ *Chapter 4: Sweat the Small Stuff*

- The bottom line to YOUR bottom line
- Common weight loss lies
- The ABCs of lifestyle change
- Get a new attitude!

Week Two:
Beneath the Surface

In This Section:

Balancing Body, Soul, and Spirit
Discovering Your True Identity
Building a Healthy Body Image

Follow-along Outline

View or listen to session two as you complete the blanks in this outline and jot down your own notes or thoughts in the margins. Then complete the workbook assignments for this week at the end of this section individually or with your group.

Balancing Body, Soul, and Spirit

For this reason I say to you, do not be worried about your life, as to what you will eat or what you will drink; nor for your body, as to what you will put on. Is not life more than food, and the body more than clothing?

Matthew 6:25

The Overextended Life

What are my excuses?

Juggling the Balls of Life

The Rubber Balls

The Glass Balls

The Expanding Balloon

Balance—What It's NOT

☐ An expertly managed lifestyle

☐ Reaching all your goals

☐ Success

☐ A stress-free life

Balance—What It IS

☐ Living with a godly perspective

☐ Making choices based on truth

☐ Doing the "right things" for the "right reasons"

☐ Leaving the results up to God

The "One Thing"

☐ Physical

☐ Material

☐ Mental

☐ Emotional

☐ Relational

☐ Spiritual

The Ultimate "One Thing"

☐ Pray as if it is the air you breathe

☐ Nourish your soul and spirit with God's Word daily

☐ Digest its truths through meditation

☐ Practice the presence of God

☐ Worship him in Spirit and in truth

Questions to Help Balance Your Life:

☐ What is the worst that can happen if I don't say "yes" to this activity or opportunity or don't get this "thing" accomplished?

☐ Will this opportunity or thing help me know and love God more?

☐ Will it help me know and love my family more?

☐ Will this help me love others more?

☐ Why else am I choosing this?

Discovering Your True Identity

Therefore if anyone is in Christ, he is a new creature; the old things passed away; behold, new things have come.

2 Corinthians 5:17

Who Are You?

What three words best describe you?

1. _____

2. _____

3. _____

What is your most important role?

Who is most important in your life?

You Are NOT:

☐ Your roles

☐ Your relationships

☐ Your behavior

What's Love Got to Do with It?

☐ Love is an incredible motivator.

☐ Pure love empowers us to obey and glorify God.

☐ It gives us a sense of significance, value, and purpose.

☐ It becomes a driving force and motivation toward healthy desires.

Building a Healthy Body Image

For man looks at the outward appearance, but the LORD looks at the heart.

1 Samuel 16:7

What Is a "Healthy" Body Image?

TRUE OR FALSE?

_____ I dislike my overall physical appearance.

_____ I'm unhappy with the size and shape of my body.

_____ I am ashamed to be seen in a swimsuit.

_____ I feel other people must think that my body is unattractive.

_____ I compare myself to others.

_____ I am self-conscious about my appearance.

_____ My body preoccupies my thinking many times during the day.

_____ I would feel okay about my body if _____.

Three things I LIKE about my physical body:

1. _____

2. _____

3. _____

Three (nonphysical) things I LIKE about myself:

1. _____

2. _____

3. _____

Three things I do NOT LIKE about myself:

1. _____

2. _____

3. _____

Tell Yourself the Truth

"With God's help, I can change my body and accept myself."
"I celebrate who I am."
"I am more than just a physical body."
"I am a wonderful creation of God."
"I can enjoy life without always thinking about how I look."
"I am focusing on my strengths more than my perceived flaws."

Personal Reflection

Answer the following questions on your own or with your group:

1. Where is your life most out of balance? What can you begin doing right now to change that?

"I will give thanks to You, for I am fearfully and wonderfully made; wonderful are Your works, and my soul knows it very well."

Psalm 139:14

2. What "one thing" would make the biggest difference in your physical dimension, and how can you begin to address that daily?

3. What "one thing" would make the biggest difference in your spiritual dimension, and how can you begin to address that daily?

4. How is your body image affecting your life, and how will you change that?

Build a Strong Spiritual Foundation

Meditate on the following Scriptures and answer the corresponding questions:

For this reason, I say to you, do not be worried about your life, as to what you will eat or what you will drink; nor for your body, as to what you will put on. Is not life more than food, and the body more than clothing?

Matthew 6:25

1. Is stress and worry impacting your life and/or lifestyle?

2. How can trusting the Lord for the details of life help you live a healthier lifestyle?

Delight yourself in the LORD; and He will give you the desires of your heart.

Psalm 37:4

1. How does delighting in the Lord impact the desires of your heart?

2. How will your desires influence your motives and/or your behavior?

Nourish Your Spirit

Life-changing spiritual victory requires daily nourishment. Continue to nourish your spirit daily in four ways:

1. Pray as if it is the air you breathe.

Pray the prayer below each day this week, surrendering every dimension of your life to the Lord.

2. Nourish your soul and spirit with God's Word daily.

Read or memorize the two Scriptures above (Matthew 6:25 and Psalm 37:4) and repeat them at least twice each day.

3. Digest its truths through meditation.

Meditate on what it means to "delight in the Lord." Imagine what your life would be like if your "one thing" was to delight in him.

4. Practice the presence of God.

Imagine eating every meal and spending every second of each day in his presence. The truth is, you ARE!

Prayer for Week Two

Heavenly Father, I am so thankful that I am a new creation in Christ. Thank you for making all things new. Please help me to not only know this truth but to believe it deep within my soul. I pray that you will also help me to identify the areas of my life that are out of balance and to surrender those areas to you. Help me learn to choose the "best" from all the "good" and to have realistic expectations about life. Lord, I celebrate that I am "fearfully and wonderfully made." I pray you will help me see my physical body from your perspective and stop comparing myself to others or to society's standard of beauty. Please remind me in my insecurity that I am the apple of your eye and beautiful inside and out. Amen.

Suggested Reading for Week Two

Read the following chapters and check off below:

☐ *Chapter 5: Balancing Body, Soul, and Spirit*

- Finding balance in your life
- What would you do if your steering wheel came off while you were driving down the freeway? Read Danna's story in this chapter!

☐ *Chapter 6: Discovering Your True Identity*

- Who are you?
- What's love got to do with it?
- Surviving an affair

☐ *Chapter 7: Building a Healthy Body Image*

- Accepting our flaws
- God's perspective on beauty and our body

Week Three:
You Are What You Think

In This Section:

Renewed Mind . . . Transformed Body

The Battle of the Flesh

Lifestyle Evaluation and Plan for Healthy Thinking

Follow-along Outline

View or listen to session three as you complete the blanks in this outline and jot down your own notes or thoughts in the margins. Then complete the workbook assignments for this week at the end of this section individually or with your group.

Renewed Mind . . . Transformed Body

Do not be conformed to this world, but be transformed by the renewing of your mind.

Romans 12:2

Your Mind—the Ultimate Computer

☐ The freeways of the mind

☐ Automatic pilot

☐ Garbage in . . . garbage out!

☐ Good stuff in . . . good stuff out!

☐ We are "leaky buckets"

☐ Erasing old tapes

☐ Building new pathways

God's Prescription for a Healthy Mind

#1 PURE THINKING

Whatever is true, whatever is noble, whatever is right, whatever is pure, whatever is lovely, whatever is admirable—if anything is excellent or praiseworthy—think about such things.

Philippians 4:8 NIV

#2 POSITIVE MODELING

Whatever you have learned or received or heard from me, or seen in me—put it into practice. And the God of peace will be with you.

Philippians 4:9 NIV

#3 PRACTICED OBEDIENCE

☐ Observation

☐ Imitation

☐ Repetition

The Power of Self-Talk

Old negative message:

"I blew it again. I'll never lose weight!"

New healthy message:

"I CAN lose weight one small step at a time!"

Old negative message:	**New healthy message:**
"I always end up quitting and never reach my goals."	"I'm not quitting. With God's help, I can reach my goals."
"I'm addicted to chocolate."	"I'm in control of every bite that goes in my mouth."
"I hate to exercise, and besides, I don't have time."	"I make time to exercise, and I love it!"

The Power of God's Word

The word of God is living and active and sharper than any two-edged sword, and piercing as far as the division of soul and spirit, of both joints and marrow, and able to judge the thoughts and intentions of the heart.

Hebrews 4:12

Your Healthy Thinking Tools

☐ The One Thing
☐ Attitudes
☐ Self-talk
☐ People power
☐ Goals
☐ Journaling
☐ Logging

Watch your thoughts; they become your words.
Watch your words; they become your actions.
Watch your actions; they become your habits.
Watch your habits; they become your character.
Watch your character; it becomes your destiny.

The Battle of the Flesh

For what I am doing, I do not understand; for I am not practicing what I would like to do, but I am doing the very thing I hate.

Romans 7:15

Choosing Your Path

☐ The path of least resistance

☐ The path of self-discipline

☐ The zigzagged path

☐ The path with real power

But I say, walk by the Spirit, and you will not carry out the desire of the flesh.

Galatians 5:16

God's Part:

- _____
- _____
- _____

Your Part:

- Draw near to God
- Abide—settle down and be at home
- Resist the devil
- Study and meditate on the Word
- Prayer
- Praise
- Thanksgiving

But the fruit of the Spirit is love, joy, peace, patience, kindness, goodness, faithfulness, gentleness, self-control; against such things there is no law.

Galatians 5:22–23

Are You Addicted to God?

1. Set your _____ on things above.

2. _____ in the Vine.

3. Walk in the _____.

4. Become "_____" to God.

5. Surrender your _____ to the Lord.

6. _____ each meal is taken with Jesus.

7. Pray for enough grace for the _____.

Starting a new program without a good evaluation is like letting the dentist drill on your teeth before he takes X-rays!

Lifestyle Evaluation and Plan for Healthy Thinking

Objective: Identify your lifestyle speed bumps
Action: Take the lifestyle self-evaluations

Truth

Ignorance is not bliss! If you don't know what the problem is, you'll have a hard time fixing it. So it's time to be totally honest with yourself.

Excuses and rationalizations undermine your achievement. Only the truth will set you free. An ancient philosopher said, "Know thyself." It wasn't bad advice.

We will begin by taking the Perspective/Healthy Thinking Self-Evaluation. This will give you a good snapshot of your current strengths and weaknesses in the area of your thinking—very important! If you don't clearly understand your weaknesses, you'll find it hard to set priorities and take action.

How to Take the Evaluation

Spend about four to five minutes on the evaluation. Base your answers on your most consistent behavior or attitudes in the past three months.

- DON'T rate yourself based on any changes you've made in the last four to six weeks.
- DO rate yourself based on your first impression and move on.
- DON'T go back and "readjust" your answers if you don't like the score!
- DO remember that this is a reality check. Just face the truth and move on.

Now it's time to face the music. Grab a pencil and be completely honest. No one has to see the results but you!

Lifestyle Evaluation: Perspective/Healthy Thinking

Based on the last three months, please rate yourself on the following statements using this scale:

0 = Almost Never   1 = Sometimes   2 = Often   3 = Always

_____ I see myself as a fully accepted and loved child of God.

_____ My choices and actions are made based on my relationship to Christ.

_____ I am thankful for the body God has given me.

_____ I honor God with my lifestyle habits.

_____ I take responsibility for my body's size, shape, and health.

_____ My attitude is this: "I am not my behavior. I am complete in Christ."

_____ I surrender my weaknesses to God and rely on his strength for the moment.

_____ My personal goals are realistic and honor God.

_____ I take realistic steps toward my goals each day.

_____ I know that with God's help, I can have a lean, healthy body.

_____ I am aware of the lies I believe about my body, looks, and health.

_____ I recognize and choose not to accept this negative thinking.

_____ I renew my mind with God's truth each day.

_____ I am a work in progress and God delights in each good step I take.

_____ Each day I choose to submit my body, mind, and spirit to God.

_____ I pray daily for God's strength to walk in the Spirit and not fulfill the desires of my flesh.

_____ Add the total of all scores.

How did you do?

Healthy Thinking Scoring:

40–48   Excellent! You have a godly perspective!

31–39   Good. Your perspective is usually working for you.

22–30   Fair. It's time to get a new focus . . . truth!

0–21   Alert! Alert! Change your perspective NOW!

Design a Healthy Thinking Success Recipe

You've evaluated your thinking. You've educated your mind. Now it's time to initiate a new plan. Trying to make too many changes all at once is unrealistic. You'll just burn out and give up. Your success depends upon your ability to prioritize your goals and design a realistic plan. If you don't take time to make these important decisions, nothing will happen. As I've said before, it has to be a plan you can live with! You are in complete control.

How to Design Your Plan

The following "Perspective/Healthy Thinking Menu" provides a list of priorities, perspectives, attitudes, and actions that will help you improve in this area. "The One Thing" category should help you identify any areas in your spiritual life that are lacking and include them as part of your personal "success recipe." Most of us definitely need to focus on identifying the lies we believe and replacing them with truth. Additionally, we need to have realistic goals coupled with the right motivations before we can realize true lifestyle victory. Reevaluating your goals and writing them down may be helpful in this process.

Based on your evaluation and gut instinct, select your top three priorities, perspective, attitude, or action that you want to improve in this lifestyle category and transfer them to the "Recipe." Then write one to three action items for each priority. An example is provided to help you.

Perspective/Healthy Thinking Menu

The One Thing

☐ I am thinking and living with God as my highest priority.
☐ I am making intimacy with the Lord my greatest desire.
☐ I need more time in the Word.

☐ I need more time in prayer.

☐ I need more time in meditation.

☐ I need more time in worship.

ATTITUDES

☐ I am building new healthy attitudes.

☐ I am securing my identity in Christ.

☐ I am developing a body image in line with God's perspective of me.

☐ I have a "small steps" perspective—small stuff counts and adds up!

SELF-TALK

☐ Identify your negative messages.

☐ Write new, positive messages.

☐ Replace negative messages with truth using trigger talk:

    ☐ Index cards   ☐ Tapes/CDs   ☐ Memorization

PEOPLE POWER

☐ I will seek out healthy role models for my lifestyle area.

☐ I will pray for a mature spiritual mentor to encourage me in my spiritual walk.

☐ I will surround myself with positive motivators who can help me along the way.

☐ I will consider a personal coach, exercise, or accountability partner.

GOAL EVALUATION

☐ I am setting realistic goals that honor God.

☐ My most important goal is:

☐ I am submitting and surrendering my goals to God.

☐ My other important goals include:

USING OTHER RESOURCES

☐ I will consider journaling for deeper insight into my habits and stumbling blocks.

☐ I will consider using the logs in this study guide for several days or weeks to help me gain insight and develop new habits.

☐ I will listen to audio resources.

☐ I will take the time to review my insights and plans as I complete this eight-week study guide.

My Perspective/Healthy Thinking Recipe

	Priority	**Action**
Example	Self-Talk	Identify the lies I believe and replace them with truth
		Listen to my self-talk CD every day
		Write out my trigger talk and post it in bathroom
#1		_____
		_____
		_____
#2		_____
		_____
		_____
#3		_____
		_____
		_____

Personal Reflection

Answer the following questions on your own or with your group:

1. What lies do you believe that are most destructive in your life?

2. How do you continue to cultivate these lies in your life?

3. Who or what else helps foster these lies?

4. What can you begin doing right now to diminish the power of these lies in your life?

5. What healthy affirmation or Scripture would help erase and replace one or more of those lies?

Build a Strong Spiritual Foundation

Meditate on the following Scripture and answer the corresponding questions:

Do not be conformed to this world, but be transformed by the renewing of your mind.

Romans 12:2

1. How do we transform our minds?

2. Write down the three ways we learn:

   a. _____

   b. _____

   c. _____

3. Who are your positive role models?

   _____

   _____

   _____

4. What do you need to spend time imitating and repeating in order to transform your thinking?

For what I am doing, I do not understand; for I am not practicing what I would like to do, but I am doing the very thing I hate.

Romans 7:15

1. The verse above was written by the apostle Paul. In your battle of the flesh, do you ever feel like Paul?

2. Does his statement encourage or discourage you? Why?

3. As you continue to read in Romans chapter 7, what hope does Paul give you for this ongoing battle?

But I say, walk by the Spirit, and you will not carry out the desire of the flesh. . . . But the fruit of the Spirit is love, joy, peace, patience, kindness, goodness, faithfulness, gentleness, self-control; against such things there is no law.

Galatians 5:16, 22–23

1. How do you know when you are walking in the Spirit?

2. What changes can you make in your life to ensure you are walking in the Spirit more often than not?

Nourish Your Spirit

Life-changing spiritual victory requires daily nourishment. Continue to nourish your spirit daily in four ways:

1. Pray as if it is the air you breathe.

This week, in addition to praying the prayer below, write your own prayer using a key Scripture that will help erase and replace at least one of the lies you are believing.

Your written prayer:

2. Nourish your soul and spirit with God's Word daily.

Memorize Romans 12:2 and Galatians 5:16 and repeat them at least twice each day.

3. Digest its truths through meditation.

Meditate on what it means to "be transformed by the renewing of your mind" (Rom. 12:2). Imagine what your life would be like if you no longer believed things which impact you negatively. What would freedom from those lies look and feel like? Imagine the victory and ask God to help your mind focus constantly on his truth.

4. Practice the presence of God.

Each time you think a negative, self-defeating thought, imagine that Jesus is standing right in front of you, his hands on each side of your face, looking intently into your eyes and saying "Stop it! I love you, and you don't need to believe these lies any longer. I have made all things new!"

Prayer for Week Three

Dear Lord, I am amazed when I consider how you designed my mind. Help me to be a better steward of my thoughts. I pray that you will bring your Word to my mind when I am believing my old lies and that your truth will erase and replace my old, destructive thinking. I choose to set my mind on things above. Please help me to address my thinking each and every day and to understand how important this principle is to every aspect of my life. May your truth set me free from bondage in all areas of unhealthy thinking and living. Teach me how to walk in the Spirit so that I will not fulfill the desires of my flesh. In Jesus's name, Amen.

Suggested Reading for Week Three

Read the following chapters and check off below:

☐ *Chapter 8: You Are What You Think*

- God's Rx for a healthy mind
- Positive modeling: observe, imitate, and repeat
- Setting godly goals
- The power of self-talk

☐ *Chapter 9: The Battle of the Flesh*

- The Holy Spirit and chocolate milk
- Choosing your path
- The enemy—Satan or me?
- Fruits of the victorious lifestyle

Week Four:
Burning Fat to the Max

In This Section:

Burning Fat to the Max

Lifestyle Fitness

Lifestyle Evaluations: Fat Management and Fitness

Follow-along Outline

View or listen to session four as you complete the blanks in this outline and jot down your own notes or thoughts in the margins. Then complete the workbook assignments for this week at the end of this section individually or with your group.

Burning Fat to the Max

Facts:

One pound of fat = 3,500 calories

One pound of muscle = 500 calories

One pound of water = 0 calories

The body is 65% water.

A 140-pound person = 91 pounds of water

One pound of fat burns 3 calories per day.

One pound of muscle burns up to 50 calories per day.

You can *eat* calories a lot faster than you can *burn* them!

Five Fat-Burning Factors:

1. Gender
2. Genetics
3. Nutrition
4. Exercise/activity
5. Muscle mass

Factors out of your control = _____ %
   Gender
   Genetics

Factors in your control = _____ %
   Lifestyle

Three Lifestyle Fat-Burning Factors

1. Nutrition
2. Exercise/activity
3. Muscle mass

NUTRITION

Fuel Storage Facts:

1 gram of carbohydrate = 4 calories

1 gram of protein = 4 calories

1 gram of fat = 9 calories

If you have 100 excess calories of:

Carbohydrate – 75% stores as fat

Protein – 60% stores as fat

Fat – 96% stores as fat!

Supporting Your "RMR" (Resting Metabolic Rate)

RMR = the number of calories you burn in 24 hours while doing
    nothing

NEVER eat less than your RMR

A very rough RMR estimate = your weight multiplied by 10*

   (*Decrease to 9 if you are very sedentary)

Eat to Burn

Eat like you have a five-gallon gas _____ in your body (fuel
    and burn all day long).

Eat for _____ energy.

Eat for _____ fat storage.

Get a reality check on _____.

EXERCISE/ACTIVITY

Move, Move, Move!

Our normal activity is NOT normal!

Your lifestyle needs to get into the act.

The #1 way to burn fat is aerobic activity.

More is not always better. Give yourself time to get in shape.

MUSCLE MASS

Notching Up Your Metabolic Engine

Fit muscles increase the fat-burning "lipolytic" enzymes.

Fit muscles burn more calories at rest.

Fit muscles increase your metabolism.

How Active Are You?

Level 0: Sedentary—rarely exercise and lifestyle is not active

Level 1: Moderate—get purposeful activity 1 to 2 times per week

Level 2: Above average—slightly active, exercise 2 to 3 times per week

Level 3: High—active lifestyle, exercise 4 to 5 times per week

Lose One Pound of Fat per Week

Determine your RMR and don't eat less!

Go to "calorie college."

Create a calorie budget.

Burn at least 500 activity calories daily.

---

500 calories per day x 7 days = 3,500 calories
3,500 calories = ONE pound of FAT!

Lifestyle Fitness

Fitness Myths

No _____ . . . no _____!

Muscle turns to _____.

You have to _____ to be fit.

Total Fitness

EXAMPLE

160-pound woman:
Daily RMR
  calorie burn: 1,600
Daily activity
  calorie burn: + 500
Total 24-hour
  calorie burn: 2,100
Daily caloric
  intake: − 1,600

NET caloric
  difference: 500

Strength

Aerobic endurance

Flexibility

STRENGTH

_____ are your body's engine.

One pound of muscle burns 50 calories per day.

Increase lipolytic, fat-burning enzymes.

You begin losing fitness in 48 to 72 hours.

SMALL STEPS to increasing your strength:

Level 1: abdominal workouts every other day.

Level 2: abdominal plus legs every other day.

Level 3: abs and legs every other day; upper body alternate days.

AEROBIC ENDURANCE

Definition of *Aerobic*: In the Presence of Oxygen

Large muscle, sustained activity

The breathing test

Target heart rate

Perceived exertion

Cardiovascular benefit

Fat-burning benefit

Warm Up
Cool Down
F.I.T.:
  Frequency
  Intensity
  Time

Benefits of Aerobic Endurance:

Lowers body fat

Improves cardiovascular fitness

Enhances immunity

Increases metabolism and energy

Releases "feel-good" hormones

FLEXIBILITY

Muscular flexibility improves:
  Posture
  Balance
  Skeletal health

Joint and muscle health

Appearance

Overall performance

SMALL STEPS to increasing your flexibility:

Level 1: warm and stretch before workouts

Level 2: stretch before and after every workout

Level 3: three or more stretch/posture sessions per week

What's Your Excuse?

I don't have _____.

I don't have _____.

I don't know _____.

I can't afford a _____.

Change Your Negative Self-Talk

Example:

Old negative message: "I can't wait until this workout is over."

New healthy message: "I am so thankful I have a body that can move!"

Example:

Old negative message: "Exercise bores me."

New healthy message: "I enjoy exercise and the way it makes me feel."

Lifestyle Evaluations: Fat Management and Fitness

Truth

Remember, ignorance is not bliss! If you don't know what the problem is, you'll have a hard time fixing it. So now is the time to be totally honest with yourself about your fitness and fat management lifestyle areas.

How to Take the Evaluations

Spend about four to five minutes on each evaluation. Base your answers on your most consistent behavior or attitudes in the past three months.

- DON'T rate yourself based on any changes you've made in the last four to six weeks.
- DO rate yourself based on your first impression and move on.
- DON'T go back and "readjust" your answers if you don't like the score!
- DO remember that this is a reality check. Just face the truth and move on.

Now it's time to face the music. Grab a pencil and be completely honest. No one has to see the results but you!

Lifestyle Evaluation: Fat Management

Based on the last three months, please rate yourself on the following statements using this scale:

0 = Almost Never   1 = Sometimes   2 = Often   3 = Always

_____ I feel in control of my food choices.

_____ I measure my size by how I look and feel, not the scale.

_____ I eat only when I'm hungry.

_____ I stop eating when I'm full.

_____ I understand why "calories count."

_____ I eat four to five small meals or snacks per day.

_____ I limit my junk food, fast food, and desserts to less than 15 percent of my diet.

_____ I am happy with my body weight.

_____ I am happy with my size and shape.

_____ I can enjoy "fun food" without feeling guilty.

_____ I think about food only when I'm hungry.

_____ I can see myself eating and living in control.

_____ I walk or get purposeful exercise at least four times per week.

_____ I am very aware of my choices and how they affect my body.

_____ I say no to the latest diets or supplements promising quick results.

_____ I know if I'm going to be lean, I have to take daily action.

_____ Add the total of all scores.

How did you do?

Fat Management Scoring:

40–48   Excellent! You've got a lean lifestyle.

31–39   Good. You're doing most things right!

22–30   Fair. It's time to take action!

0–21   Poor. Start with one step at a time.

Lifestyle Evaluation: Fitness

Based on the last three months, please rate yourself on the following statements using this scale:

0 = Almost Never   1 = Sometimes   2 = Often   3 = Always

_____ I crave activity and find ways to move more each day.

_____ I enjoy exercise and how it makes my body feel.

_____ I have high energy to do all the things I want and need to do.

_____ I make exercise and activity a priority in my life.

_____ I understand the need for aerobic, strength, and flexibility training.

_____ I engage in aerobic activity four or more times per week.

_____ I take the stairs or park far away whenever I can.

_____ I monitor my heart rate and know I am exercising safely.

_____ I am injury-free and able to engage in most activities freely.

_____ Being healthy and fit is important to me.

_____ I listen to my body and know what it needs.

_____ I wear shoes that are appropriate and of good quality for exercise.

_____ I have a very active life and am moving throughout the day.

_____ I work out my major muscle groups two to three times each week.

_____ I can easily touch my toes without bending my knees.

_____ I maintain strong abdominal muscles.

_____ Add the total of all scores.

How did you do?

Fitness Scoring:

40–51   Excellent! You're a fit machine!

31–39   Good. Stay consistent!

22–30   Fair. Use it or lose it!

0–21   Poor. Take one small step and start moving!

Design a Fat Management Success Recipe

You've evaluated your lifestyle. You've educated your mind. Now it's time to initiate a new plan. Trying to make too many changes all at once is unrealistic. You'll just burn out and give up. Your success depends upon your ability to prioritize your goals and design a realistic plan. If you don't take time to make these important decisions, nothing will happen. As I've said before, it has to be a plan you can live with! You are in complete control.

HOW TO DESIGN YOUR PLAN

The following Fat Management Menu provides a list of things you can do to improve in this area. Based on your evaluation, select your top three priorities in this lifestyle category and transfer them to the recipe page. Then write one to three action items for each priority. An example is provided to help you.

Fat Management Menu

Increase Your Daily Calorie Burn

☐ Aerobic activity is best

☐ An active lifestyle makes a difference

☐ Wear Caltrac—your personal activity coach

Decrease Your Daily Calorie Intake

☐ Read labels

☐ Find enjoyable substitutions

☐ Count calories for absolute truth

☐ Keep a food diary

☐ Use portion control

☐ Plan your snacks

☐ Shop for success

☐ Cut your losses

Get a Handle on Emotional Eating

☐ Identify your triggers

☐ Create new habits

☐ Tune into the hunger scale

☐ Legalize foods

☐ Discard old diet attitudes

☐ Learn to cut your losses

Increase Your Energy and Metabolism

☐ Practice the NutriMax Six (see Nutrition Menu)

☐ Never eat less than your RMR!

☐ Fuel and burn all day long

Practice Healthy Thinking

☐ Identify your lies.

☐ Rewrite your self-talk.

☐ Listen to your tapes.

☐ Practice trigger talk whenever possible—in the car, on the potty, everywhere!

My Fat Management Recipe

	Priority	Action
Example	Decrease intake	Count calories for a one-month reality check
		Pre-package healthy snacks to take with me
		Practice portion control—use smaller plate
#1		_____
		_____
		_____
#2		_____
		_____
		_____
#3		_____
		_____
		_____

Design a Fitness Success Recipe

Now it's time to do the same thing in your lifestyle fitness category. You know the drill . . . pick three priorities and write an action plan. Let's get started.

Fitness Menu

Aerobic Fitness: The Ultimate Calorie Burn

☐ Level 1: 15 to 20 minutes 3 times per week

☐ Level 2: 20 to 30 minutes 5 times per week

☐ Level 3: 30+ minutes 6 to 7 times per week

Strength and Toning: Tuning Your Body's Engine

☐ Level 1: abdominal workouts every other day

☐ Level 2: abdominal plus leg toning every other day

☐ Level 3: add upper body 2–3 times per week, plus abs and legs every other day

Flexibility: Posture and Prevention

☐ Level 1: "Warm" and stretch tight muscles before workouts

☐ Level 2: Stretch before and after every workout

☐ Level 3: Three or more stretch and posture sessions per week

The Lifestyle: Movin' and Groovin'

☐ All activity counts, so move, move, move!

☐ Never sit if you can stand

☐ Never stand when you can walk

Advanced Fitness

☐ Cross training to enhance overall fitness

☐ Interval training for variety and strength

☐ Specific sport training and strengthening

☐ Distance running or competitive training

Aches, Pains, and Limitations

☐ Take care of "problems" first

☐ Prevention is essential—broken bodies slow you down!

☐ Seek the advice of professionals and follow that advice!

My Fitness Recipe

Priority	Action
#1	
#2	
#3	

How Long Does It Take to Burn 100 Calories?

Activity	Duration	Calories Burned
Biking	15 min	96
In-line skating	15 min	104
Jogging (10 min/mile)	10 min	113
Jumping rope	10 min	100
Walking (15 min/mile)	15 min	113

Estimates based on a 130-pound female. The more you weigh, the more you'll burn per minute.

Recommended Fitness Resources

☐ Total body home fitness equipment: Total Gym www.totalgym .com

☐ Exercise videotapes by Karen Voight and Kathy Smith

☐ Posture/pain resource: www.egoscue.com

Personal Reflection

Answer the following questions on your own or with your group:

1. What is the most important principle you have learned about how your body burns fat, and how will you apply it to your life?

2. What did your Fat Management evaluation reveal about your weaknesses in this area?

3. What is your greatest challenge in the area of lifestyle fitness, and how will you address that challenge?

4. How does your attitude and self-talk impact your fat management and fitness issues?

Build a Strong Spiritual Foundation

Meditate on the following Scripture and answer the corresponding questions:

On the other hand, discipline yourself for the purpose of godliness; for bodily discipline is only of little profit, but godliness is profitable for all things, since it holds promise for the present life and also for the life to come.

1 Timothy 4:7–8

1. Does the fact that the apostle Paul says bodily discipline is only of little profit mean that we should disregard it?

2. How can physical discipline help us build mental and spiritual discipline?

3. Do you think the people of Paul's day had to work at being lean and fit?

4. How will you find balance between the disciplines of body, soul, and spirit?

Nourish Your Spirit

Life-changing spiritual victory requires daily nourishment. Continue to nourish your spirit daily in four ways:

1. Pray as if it is the air you breathe.

This week, spend some time praising the Lord for the blessings of your body. Thank him if you are able to walk or do other activities without too much difficulty. Ask him to help you worship him and celebrate this great gift by moving more and getting more physically fit.

2. Nourish your soul and spirit with God's Word daily.

Before eating too many calories . . . feed yourself truth from God's Word. Feast on his powerful principles and let it transform you from the inside out.

3. Digest its truths through meditation.

Imagine and meditate on how you can glorify God by living a victorious lifestyle—one that increases your health, vitality, and passion for ministry.

4. Practice the presence of God.

As you eat and burn like a car with a five-gallon tank, walk or run to maximize fat burning, or engage in strength training or flexibility exercises, imagine that the Lord is your workout partner. Just as we are encouraged by Paul to "work as unto the Lord" (see Col. 3:23), why not "work out as unto the Lord" as well?

Prayer for Week Four

Heavenly Father, thank you for my body. Please forgive me for not caring for it as a precious gift from you. I desire to honor you in my body by eating, moving, and living in ways that enhance my health and energy. Please help me to have a godly desire that pursues physical fitness without diminishing my commitment to spiritual fitness. Lord, I need to find the balance that only you can give. Show me how to transform my lifestyle to your glory. Amen.

Suggested Reading for Week Four

Read the following chapters and check off below:

☐ *Chapter 12: Burning Fat to the Max*

- Finding your "one thing" for burning fat
- The bottom line to your bottom line
- Your body's three fuel sources
- Five fat-burning factors
- From knowledge to action in four steps

☐ *Chapter 16: Use It or Lose It . . . Lifestyle Fitness*

- How to get started safely
- Danna's TV workout

Week Five:
You Are What You Eat

In This Section:

Nutritional Basics

The NutriMax Six

The NutriZap Four

Lifestyle Evaluation: Nutrition

Follow-along Outline

View or listen to session five as you complete the blanks in this outline and jot down your own notes or thoughts in the margins. Then complete the workbook assignments for this week at the end of this section individually or with your group.

Nutritional Basics

Your diet each day is composed of carbohydrates, protein, and fat. A common question is how much of each fuel source a person should eat. These are the recommended ranges:

Percentage of total calories:

Carbohydrates	45–60%
Proteins	15–30%
Fats	15–30%

Grams (based on 2,000 calorie diet):

Carbohydrates	220–300 grams
Proteins	75–150 grams
Fats	33–55 grams

The NutriMax Six

NutriMax #1: Water

A quart low and running on steam

Wasted _____ – wasted _____

Headaches and hunger

The caffeine/water facts

Get the plastic out (don't refill plastic water bottles!)

NutriMax #2: Plant Foods

The "real" carbohydrates

Antioxidant power

Phytochemicals

Fiber's many roles

Enzymes for life

NutriMax #3: Protein

How much is enough?

Where's the beef?

Fish facts

Other sources

Blood sugar balance

NutriMax #4: Essential Fats

The good

The essential

The bad

The ugly

NutriMax #5: Vital Vitamins

Danna's Top-Ten Supplements List

1. High-potency vitamin-mineral complex
2. Super green foods
3. Essential fatty acids
4. Vitamin C
5. Garlic
6. Calcium/magnesium
7. Vitamin E
8. Ginkgo Biloba
9. Green tea
10. Milk thistle

NutriMax #6: Vitamins Z and X

Vitamin Z: _____ – you can't live without it!

Vitamin X: _____ – you need it even if you don't like it!

The NutriZap Four

#1   Sugar

#2   White Flour

#3   Caffeine

#4   Artificial Sweeteners

   Saccharin

   Aspartame

   Splenda

Healthy alternatives:

Stevia: see www.mdvventures.com

Xylitol: see www.globalsweet.com

Lo Han: see www.easymuscle.com

Learn to Read Labels

How many portions?

How big are they?

How many calories?

How much fat and what kind?

How much protein?

How much fiber?

What's the nutritional value?

Is this food worth the "cost"?

Small Steps Add Up!

A 20 percent improvement *for a lifetime* is better than a 100 percent improvement for a few weeks or months!

Add more natural foods.

Eat fewer packaged products.

Keep it balanced.

Remember . . . you ARE what you eat!

Lifestyle Evaluation: Nutrition

How to Take the Evaluation

Spend about four to five minutes on the evaluation. Base your answers on your most consistent behavior or attitudes in the past three months.

- DON'T rate yourself based on any changes you've made in the last four to six weeks.
- DO rate yourself based on your first impression and move on.

- DON'T go back and "readjust" your answers if you don't like the score!

- DO remember that this is a reality check. Just face the truth and move on.

Now it's time to face the music. Grab a pencil and be completely honest. No one has to see the results but you!

Lifestyle Evaluation: Nutrition

Based on the last three months, please rate yourself on the following statements using this scale:

0 = Never or Don't Know   1 = Sometimes   2 = Often   3 = Always

_____ I think about what I eat and how it impacts my health.

_____ I have high energy to do all the things I want and need to do.

_____ I read labels and choose many foods based on that information.

_____ I eat 2 to 3 servings of fruit each day.

_____ I eat 3 to 4 servings of vegetables each day.

_____ I choose whole grain products over more processed foods.

_____ I know how much fiber I'm eating daily.

_____ I drink 10 to 12 glasses of water daily.

_____ I eat breakfast every day.

_____ I eat a good source of protein at breakfast.

_____ I choose and eat lean protein with my lunch.

_____ I limit my "empty" calories to less than 15 percent of my total diet.

_____ I limit caffeine, other stimulants, and over-the-counter diet aids.

_____ I take a multi-vitamin supplement daily.

_____ I take an antioxidant supplement daily.

_____ I choose "healthy" fats in my diet like olive or Canola oil.

_____ Add the total of all scores.

How did you do?

Nutrition Scoring:

40–48   Excellent! Your body loves you!

31–39   Good. You're on the right track.

22–30   Fair. It's time to try a little more high-octane fuel.

0–21   Poor. Your body's crying "Help!"

Design a Nutrition Success Recipe

Now that you've evaluated your nutrition and educated your mind, it's time to initiate a new plan. If you don't take time to make these important decisions, nothing will happen. Your success depends upon your ability to prioritize your goals, design a realistic plan, and surrender it daily to God. As I've said before, it has to be a plan you can live with! You are in complete control. This is a very important category and an example is provided to help you.

Remember, you build a completely new body every seven years, including your skeleton. It can only be as strong as the supplies you give it to work with. So as you make decisions about how you will eat and live for a lifetime, keep in mind that you can't build a brick house out of straw, nor can you build a healthy body out of sugar!

Example: "My Nutrition Recipe"

	Priority	Action
#1	Drink more water	Drink with meals
		Carry bottle with me
#2	Eat more veggies	Keep stocked up – make it easy
		Order more salads

	Priority	**Action**
#3	Less poison!	Artificial sweeteners – limit to 2 or 3 servings per week
		Decrease caffeine
		Fast food only once per week
#4	Increase fiber	Start with high fiber and protein breakfast
		Add beans and read labels for fiber content

Nutrition Menu

Wonderful Water

☐ 8 to 12 glasses per day

☐ Carry water with you

☐ Limit caffeinated beverages

Fiber-Rich Fruits

☐ 3 to 4 fruits per day (most servings equal ½ cup)

☐ Whole fruits instead of juice

☐ Variety is important

Fiber-Rich Veggies

☐ 4 to 5 veggies per day (most servings equal ½ cup)

☐ Quality counts . . . French fries don't!

☐ Frozen is as good as fresh

Quality Carbos

☐ Beans, bran, and "brown"

☐ White bagels and pretzels don't count

☐ Whole grain on the label is the key

☐ Nuts in moderation

Powerful Proteins

☐ Always with breakfast and lunch

☐ Healthy shakes and bars

☐ Keep stocked with easy choices

Fabulous Fats—Omegas Rule!

☐ Increase Omega 3's the most—fish, flaxseed, walnuts

☐ Omega 6's—keep vegetable oils to a bare minimum

☐ Omega 9's—choose olive oil over vegetable oil

☐ Nuts are okay—watch the calories

☐ Keep saturated fat to 10 percent of total fat max!

Vital Vitamins

☐ Fill in your nutritional gaps

☐ Multi-vitamin and mineral in two doses

☐ Antioxidants to fight free radicals

☐ Choose five from the top-ten list and be consistent

Fuel and Burn

☐ Start with breakfast

☐ Eat like a car with a five-gallon tank

☐ Stop when you're full

☐ Eat lighter at night

Pick Your "Poisons"

☐ Limit junk food and chemicals

☐ Fun food: no more than 15 percent

☐ Artificial sweeteners: less than 3 servings per week

☐ Limit sugar and caffeine

My Nutrition Recipe

	Priority	Action
#1		
#2		
#3		
#4		

Personal Reflection

Answer the following questions on your own or with your group:

1. How are you doing? You've been working on your new lifestyle for a few weeks now. What do your lifestyle behaviors say about the changes you are (or aren't) making in the following areas:

   ☐ The quality of my nutrition says:
   ☐ The amount of food I eat says:
   ☐ The way I move and exercise says:
   ☐ The way I relax and sleep says:
   ☐ The way I respond to stress or worry says:

2. How do you feel about your progress thus far?

3. What changes or help will you pursue to continue to change your attitudes and behavior?

Nourish Your Spirit

Meditate on the following Scripture and answer the corresponding questions:

Whether, then, you eat or drink or whatever you do, do all to the glory of God.

1 Corinthians 10:31

1. Try to imagine every meal or snack you eat as if you are enjoying it with the Lord. How would that change your behavior?

2. How do we influence our motives and attitudes about food and our habits so that they do glorify God?

3. Imagine every food and drink that you ingest either building up your body or diminishing your health. Do we glorify God when we eat empty calories or unhealthy foods in excess?

Life-changing spiritual victory requires daily nourishment. Continue to nourish your spirit daily in four ways:

1. Pray as if it is the air you breathe.

Include in your prayers this week a focus on thankfulness for the incredible gift of taste and smell. Praise God for his wonderful provision of food to nourish our bodies. Surrender your battle with food to the Lord and ask him to transform your thinking about food so that you eat to live rather than "live to eat," if that is a challenge for you. Ask him to help you see your body from the inside out and come to a full realization that what you eat becomes your new body each day, week, month, and year.

2. Nourish your soul and spirit with God's Word daily.

Look back at the Scriptures that have been used so far in this program and in this workbook, and pick one or two that you believe best feed your soul in the area of your lifestyle. Memorize those and study them in the context of their complete chapter for greater understanding.

3. Digest its truths through meditation.

Meditate on one or more of those verses this week. Ask the Lord to illuminate and animate those truths in your mind and spirit as you digest them more fully and allow them to transform your life.

4. Practice the presence of God.

Continue to focus on seeing the Lord with you at every meal and even as you sometimes struggle with the temptation of food. Realize his unconditional love for you and his desire to help you grow in victory.

Prayer for Week Five

Father God, I am so thankful that you have given me all I need to eat and live. I am thankful for the wonder of my five senses and for the great pleasure that smell and taste bring. I pray that I would not misuse this gift and eat more than my body needs or take in too many empty calories or foods that cause my body damage. Help me to see food as a source of nutrition first and joy second. Help me to enjoy and celebrate foods the way you originally made them. I choose to present my body as a living sacrifice to you. Be glorified in my habits and health. Amen.

Suggested Reading for Week Five

Read the following chapter and check off below:

☐ *Chapter 13: You Are What You Eat*

This chapter is full of great nutritional information. Because everyone wants to know what and how to eat, it's important material. Here you'll learn my basic philosophy and read in-depth teaching about the NutriMax Six, the NutriZap Four, fiber, protein, carbos, fats, water, and more!

☐ *Extra Assignment*

Buy a "food counts" book that includes fiber, calories, protein, carbohydrate, and fat content information. You'll find many choices on the bookstore shelves. One I have used over the years is *The Complete Book of Food Counts* by Corrine Netzer. Calorie counting may seem like drudgery, but you only need to do it for about a month to reap the benefit for life. Go to calorie college and get a reality check on what you're really eating. Write down your regular meals and calculate the calories and nutritional value. We're creatures of habit and tend to eat a lot of the same things most of the time. This exercise is a real eye-opener and will give you valuable insight as you continue your lifestyle journey.

Week Six:
You Are What You Don't Eat

In This Section:

You Are What You Don't Eat
Overcoming Emotional Eating

Follow-along Outline

View or listen to session six as you complete the blanks in this outline and jot down your own notes or thoughts in the margins. Then complete the workbook assignments for this week at the end of this section individually or with your group.

You Are What You Don't Eat

Do You Eat Only When You Are Hungry?

No temptation has overtaken you but such as is common to man; and God is faithful, who will not allow you to be tempted beyond what you are able, but with the temptation will provide the way of escape also, so that you will be able to endure it. Therefore, my beloved, flee from idolatry.

1 Corinthians 10:13–14

Grumbling in the Wilderness

Who will give us meat to eat? We remember the fish, which we used to eat free in Egypt, the cucumbers and the melons and the leeks and the onions and the garlic, but now our appetite is gone. There is nothing at all to look at except this manna.

Numbers 11:4–6

Overcoming Emotional Eating

Legalize food

Tune in to the hunger scale

Identify emotional eating triggers

Change your self-talk

Energize for self-control

Legalize Food

There are no "_____" foods.

I can eat this food _____.

So I don't have to eat it _____.

And I don't have to eat it _____.

I'm putting dangerous foods "_____."

I'm practicing "_____."

The Hunger Scale

At 1: I am "starving"!

At 2: I'm slightly hungry.

At 3: I feel neutral.

At 4: I'm physically satisfied.

At 5: I'm "Thanksgiving" full.

When You Feel like Eating, Ask Yourself . . .

☐ Am I really hungry?

☐ If not, what's really going on?

☐ And what should I do instead? Sleep?

☐ If I am hungry, what will satisfy me?

Change Your Self-Talk

From:

"I can't stop eating until I'm overstuffed. My appetite is out of control."

To:

"I am in control of my appetite and cannot stand feeling full. It is absolutely unbearable, so I never do it!"

Identify Emotional Eating Triggers

THE EVENT-FOOD CONNECTION

☐ Christmas

☐ Birthday parties

☐ Ball games

☐ The movies

☐ Television

☐ Working at your desk

☐ Riding in the car

HALT! ARE YOU:

☐ Hungry?

☐ Angry?

☐ Lonely?

☐ Tired?

Energize for Self-Control

The Positive Energy Cycle

☐ Get adequate sleep

☐ Manage stress

☐ Eat and drink for maximum energy

☐ Exercise for maximum energy

Five Tips for Reducing Calories

#1 DAYTIME EATING

If most people simply ate one-half their usual volume of food from 6 p.m. until bedtime, they would _____.

#2 SUBSTITUTION

Find _____ and _____ options that still taste good!

Follow the 80% satisfaction rule.

#3 MEAL REPLACEMENTS

Find a _____, _____, or _____ _____ that you like for busy days or "emergencies."

#4 PORTION CONTROL

Quit the "clean plate club."

Eat the same . . . just eat less!

Use a _____ plate.

#5 CALORIES

Get a good "food counts" book.

Learn to conceptualize calories.

_____ your favorite foods.

If it's worth eating, it's worth counting.

Your body is a perfect calorie counting machine.

Go to "_____   _____" for one month.

Hints on Conceptualizing Calories

Check out the labels on frozen foods.

Get familiar with serving sizes.

When in doubt, measure.

Err conservatively—count HIGH!

Be honest with yourself.

Equate Serving Sizes with Everyday Items

A deck of cards = 3 ounces of meat

Your fist = 1 cup of rice or potatoes

Your thumb = 1 ounce of cheese or candy

Decrease Your Caloric Intake

Learn to:

- _____
- _____
- _____
- _____
- _____

Words for the Walk

Physical Checkpoints

Find creative ways to eat fewer calories daily.

Develop a more active lifestyle.

Eat for maximum energy and health.

Soul Checkpoints

Discover the lies you believe.

Replace lies with truth.

Observe, imitate, and repeat healthy thinking and living.

Get and be an excellent role model.

Spiritual Checkpoints

Pray as if it is the air you breathe.

Feed your soul with God's Word.

Digest its truth through meditation.

Practice the presence of God.

Personal Reflection

Answer the following questions on your own or with your group:

1. What three changes would make the biggest difference in your nutrition if you chose to implement them on a daily basis?

   a. _____

   b. _____

   c. _____

2. What are your biggest emotional eating triggers?

3. What principles, Scriptures, or techniques will you use to address those triggers?

4. Choose three to four calorie-cutting strategies that you will try to implement this week and write them here.

a. _____

b. _____

c. _____

d. _____

Build a Strong Spiritual Foundation

Meditate on the following Scripture and answer the corresponding questions:

All things are lawful for me, but not all things are profitable. All things are lawful for me, but I will not be mastered by anything. Food is for the stomach and the stomach is for food, but God will do away with both of them.

1 Corinthians 6:12–13

1. If everything is lawful or permissible, how do you make the right choices?

2. Do you feel like anything in your life has mastery over you? If so, what is it?

3. Why does Paul tell us that God will do away with both food and the stomach?

4. How do we get ourselves to choose God's glorification instead of our immediate gratification?

No temptation has overtaken you but such as is common to man; and God is faithful, who will not allow you to be tempted beyond what you are able, but with the temptation will provide the way of escape also, so that you will be able to endure it. Therefore, my beloved, flee from idolatry.

1 Corinthians 10:13–14

1. Is food an idol in your life, and if so, how?

2. How can you change that, and how can you "flee" from that form of idolatry?

Abide in Me, and I in you. As the branch cannot bear fruit of itself unless it abides in the vine, so neither can you unless you abide in Me. I am the vine, you are the branches; he who abides in Me and I in him, he bears much fruit, for apart from Me you can do nothing. . . . If you abide in Me, and My words abide in you, ask whatever you wish, and it will be done for you. My Father is glorified by this, that you bear much fruit, and so prove to be My disciples.

John 15:4–5, 7–8

1. What do you think it means to "abide" in Christ?

2. Do you ever experience times when you feel "disconnected" from him?

3. What kind of "fruit" do we bear when we abide?

Nourish Your Spirit

Life-changing spiritual victory requires daily nourishment. Continue to nourish your spirit daily in four ways:

1. Pray as if it is the air you breathe.

Choose one or two of the Scriptures in this week's Build a Strong Spiritual Foundation section and personalize them in a prayer to the Lord. Ask him to show you how to flee the idolatry of food. Focus on how much more satisfying and enriching the power of prayer is than the desires of the flesh. Ask that he transform your mind to truly believe that truth.

2. Nourish your soul and spirit with God's Word daily.

Study the areas of your greatest weaknesses and surrender your heart and mind in the process, asking God to reveal his truth to you in a very personal way. Look for practical ways to implement these truths in your life.

3. Digest its truths through meditation.

Meditate on the Scriptures you are praying this week. Say them over and over. See yourself submitting to those truths. Imagine the glory you bring to God when you surrender your battle to him and lift your praises to him as he gives you victory in your struggles.

4. Practice the presence of God.

One of the hardest things to do is to imagine God with you when you are stumbling with temptation or sin. And the truth is, *he is*! So this week imagine his presence. And rather than respond in shame, respond in surrender and with petitions for his divine intervention in the midst of trials.

Prayer for Week Six

Heavenly Father, I am so thankful that you love me for who I am in Christ rather than for how I behave. I delight to do your will, Lord. Please help me to run to you, rather than from you, in the midst of my temptations. Show me where I idolize food, comfort, or other things over you. Show me the "way of escape" and lead me down the path of the Spirit where I can experience the fruit of the Spirit on a daily basis. In Jesus's name, Amen.

Suggested Reading for Week Six

Read the following chapters and check off below:

☐ *Chapter 10: Overcoming Emotional Eating*

- Do you live to eat?
- What does healthy eating look like?
- Legalizing food
- Getting in tune with your hunger
- Identifying your eating triggers

☐ *Chapter 14: You Are What You Don't Eat*

- "Oh my goodness, that's why I'm fat!" exclaimed Pamela
- What lifestyle revelations have you had?
- Effective calorie control without dieting
- Meal planning, dining strategically, and surviving special occasions
- Shopping for success
- 52 calorie-busting ideas

☐ Chapter 17: Words for the Walk

Congratulations! You've made it to the last chapter of the book. The section titles are "Victory at Last" and "The Joy Factor." It's short but important. Continued blessings on your *Scale Down* journey.

I also recommend the following two books:

- *Idols of the Heart* by Elyse Fitzpatrick
- *Classic Christianity* by Bob George

Week Seven:
Healthy Eating and Cooking Ideas

In This Section:

Keys to Calorie Control

Healthy Eating and Cooking Ideas

Favorite Recipes

Whether you are participating in a group or going through this program alone, now is the time to begin to seriously implement many of the nutritional concepts you've been learning. For this reason, I have taken many of the expanded nutritional concepts from the book that were not covered in the CD or DVD program and reintroduced them here for your convenience.

I have also added extra ideas and recipes to foster more success. In addition, I want to point out a very helpful website that you may want to visit. It is: www.caloriecounter.com. When reading through this section, take a highlighter or red pen and mark the ideas that appeal to you. Then put those items on your shopping list.

Be Nutritionally Prepared

As I write this week's study information, I am on a plane to Virginia Beach, Virginia, to appear on *The 700 Club* with Pat Robertson and talk about the concepts from *Scale Down*. Can you guess what this particular airline is serving on our almost five-hour flight across the country? Here goes.

First, we are offered an assortment of beverages (I already had a bottle of water with my two packets of "EmergenC" mixed in, so I opted for hot water to make my own tea). To complement our beverage, we get a package of vanilla wafers that have 200 calories and not even a smidge of protein or fiber. I was so glad I brought a protein energy bar since my plane left at 7:45 a.m. and I didn't have time for breakfast before leaving.

Then, an hour later, we were promised a more substantial snack box. I thought perhaps they'd include an apple and some cheese. The closest we got to cheese was the Cheese Whiz–type filling in the Ritz crackers. To complement all the carbos, we got a package of Oreos and some gummie-like Jell-O candies.

Can you say "blood sugar crisis"? The good news is, after thirty minutes the plane is very quiet. Everyone who ate that snack is sleeping it off. Thank goodness they did give me one half ounce of peanuts. I'll be a little hungry when I hit my destination but still high-energy and ready for a "real" meal.

One of the key things you've been learning is that to have lifestyle victory and to avoid blood sugar crashes, you need to *be prepared*. So dig into this information and put some of it into action. And the next time you're a mile high on a nutritionally challenged airline, you'll be ready!

Keys to Calorie Control

Planning for Success

Your success in developing a healthy approach to cutting calories depends on your willingness to change your old ways of doing things and plan, plan, plan. The best way to avoid an eating disaster is to be prepared! The following ideas will ensure you are prepared for anything!

- Plan all meals beforehand
- Dine out strategically and know your options
- Learn how to survive special occasions
- Practice "calorie-busting"
- Shop for success

Meal Planning

It will take a little time for you to develop a lifestyle of eating that is both satisfying and effective in helping you burn off excess fat. No single plan will work for everyone. You must plan your eating based on your likes, dislikes, lifestyle, and objectives.

Each time you decide to have a meal or snack, you must decide what choices will best meet all your objectives. The more satisfied you are after a meal, the better the chance you will not overeat later. Consider these factors:

- What sounds good?
- How hungry am I?
- How many calories have I burned?
- How many calories will I burn?
- How many calories can I afford to eat?
- What do I feel like eating right now?
- Will it give me adequate protein and fiber to stabilize my blood sugar?

PLAN WITH A PURPOSE

Most people find that they are satisfied with one or two main breakfast options, several lunch choices, and a wide variety at dinner. To help you get your lifestyle in check, try to determine two to three healthy breakfasts, three to four lunch choices, and five to six dinner options that fit with your personal tastes and move you toward your lifestyle goals. Write these down in a notebook or on index cards and rotate the choices over the next several weeks. Make sure that you are always getting a good source of protein and fiber at breakfast and lunch. And, of course, dinner is the meal that needs to be smallest, so decrease your portions and eliminate the "unnecessary" such as bread. Keep snacks to 100 to 200 calories maximum. Whenever possible, try to find foods that have some fiber or protein as well to help stabilize your blood sugar.

The following ideas may help you make better meal and snack choices. You don't have to write out detailed eating plans to lose excess fat, but you do need to be purposeful, wise, and committed to eating for maximum energy and never taking in more calories than you burn.

BREAKFAST

As you learned in the NutriMax Six, breakfast is the meal that "jump-starts" your metabolism for the day. It's important to fuel up within the first two hours of waking, even if you don't feel hungry. In fact, some studies indicate that eating breakfast can increase your metabolism by up to 10 percent! Try to include protein and fiber with each meal. Avoid simple sugars and caffeine early in the day to ensure a stable blood sugar.

LUNCH

Lunch should be your most substantial meal. It needs to sustain you through your busy day. It will impact your hunger in those dangerous hours in the evening. Lunch is an excellent time to include a little more protein in your diet through lean poultry and fish or lots of beans and legumes. Planning will ensure you make healthy choices. Include leftovers from previous dinners or choices from healthy restaurants.

SNACK OPTIONS

Remember it's best to fuel and burn with frequent, small meals or snacks all day long for maximum energy. It's good to always have healthy snack options with you, such as a sturdy piece of fruit like an orange or apple and a bottle of water, for a quick snack when you're on the go. I also like good energy bars with adequate protein and a little fat.

They satisfy my hunger and sweet cravings, and the protein stabilizes my blood sugar. The important thing is to avoid reaching "1" on the hunger scale. Another good strategy is to have "pre-portioned" baggies or containers with nuts, dried fruit, or other snacks that are quickly satisfying. But if not pre-measured, many snacks turn into excess calories and ultimately excess fat.

DINNER OPTIONS

In our culture, dinner has traditionally been our main meal. But think about it: in reality, you have no need to fuel up for rest, relaxation, or sleep. Dinner should be taken as early in the evening as possible and kept fairly light. Consider it roughly one-fifth of your daily calories or a maximum of about 400 to 500 calories on an active day. If you are an evening "snacker," make dinner even lighter.

TAKE THE CHALLENGE AND LOSE A POUND A WEEK!

I personally believe that most people would lose weight very easily if they would simply cut in half the amount of calories they eat in the last four hours of each day. For most, that would be at least 500 calories per day. That is one pound of fat per week and 52 pounds in a year. Make sense? Why not test my theory on yourself?

You'll find many healthy food suggestions in this section but not very extensive menu plans. That is because I do not believe that telling people exactly how to eat is a good long-term plan for losing weight and keeping it off. You are highly unlikely to eat based on prepared meal plans for the rest of your life. My purpose is to educate you so that you can make food choices that will work for you. Make your choices based on the energy, body size, and lifestyle you desire.

KEEP IT SIMPLE

Keep your healthy eating as simple as possible to ensure success. Don't underestimate the very simple yet profound principle I have been teaching you from day one: eat a little less and burn a little more each and every day. And when you find yourself in circumstances where you have little or no choice, remember that the very simple technique of portion control is always a helpful tool.

Shopping for Success

To keep your calories under control, you must have a wide variety of excellent choices always at hand. Plan a day when you can spend an extra thirty or forty minutes in the grocery store "exploring." You will be amazed at some of the fantastic new foods that are great alternatives to some of the more fattening old favorites. Shop with a mission and make sure you never enter a grocery store hungry! Reading labels accurately is also very important. *Never* buy anything in a bag, can, or box without reading the label first!

CREATE A SHOPPING LIST

Try to have a working grocery list with you at all times. When you think of an item that will help you refine your lifestyle, add it to the list. So do you have a piece of paper handy? You'll probably find a few items you'll want to put on your list in the next several pages!

The next time you need to visit the store, shop the perimeter *first*, focusing on fresh fruits, veggies, and healthy protein choices as the staple of your diet. Then you can move on to finding an assortment of healthy packaged and convenience food choices. Make sure you have something in each of the following categories:

- Fast breakfast, lunch, and dinner options for when time is an issue
- Fruits and veggies that need little preparation (baby carrots, apples, bananas)
- Healthy and quick snacks or meal replacements (Balance bars, nuts, canned soup)
- Purified, filtered, or bottled water (always)
- Calorie/portion controlled treats (low fat ice cream bars, graham crackers, and healthy frozen meals)

Dining Out Strategically

Dining out doesn't need to be an exercise in frustration where you feel like you've completely lost control. By understanding nutrition basics, you can eat almost anywhere healthfully. Don't be afraid to ask for what you want; you are the customer.

REVIEW RESTAURANT CHOICES

Write down all the restaurants you visit at least once each month. Determine what you believe to be the best choices and order those. Take the time to go to their websites for nutritional information, or ask for their information the next time you are there. Just be sure and check it out *before* you order, or you could get an upset stomach! A great resource is the book *Eating Out Food Counter* by Annette Natow and Jo-Ann Heslin.

9 WAYS TO DINE OUT STRATEGICALLY

1. Decide beforehand what kind of food choices you will make.
2. Be assertive when requesting your food servings and preparation.
3. Consider sharing or ordering half-portions.
4. Ask how much fat is used in preparation and, if necessary, ask for it to be reduced.
5. Have the waiter remove your plate as soon as you feel full.
6. Never go out when you're a "1" on the hunger scale.
7. Avoid the words *fried, breaded, creamed, au gratin,* and *à la mode!*
8. Remember that white sauces are always richer than red.
9. Ask for your salad tossed with a half portion of salad dressing or pasta with half the sauce.

MOVE ON WHEN YOU BLOW IT

When you eat too much or make poor choices, don't sabotage your entire day (or week) by caving in emotionally. Make a mental note of how uncomfortable you feel when you've eaten too much or how badly you feel when your energy plummets. Remind yourself how great you feel when you make better choices. Then . . . GET OVER IT! If we simply learn to cut our losses and get back on track, the blowouts will rarely have a huge impact.

Surviving Special Occasions

Holidays and special occasions almost always include high-calorie foods. Whenever you attend a party or special event, several strategies can help you take control of your calorie intake. First, never, never starve yourself beforehand. That is a sure way to increase the chance of a blowout! Here are seven more strategies for surviving special occasions:

1. Start the day with breakfast, and practice the NutriMax Six. High energy means less cravings!
2. Offer to bring a low-calorie snack or contribution to the meal.
3. Brush your teeth just before the event. Food just doesn't taste as good right after brushing.
4. At parties, stand away from the goodies and focus on socializing.
5. Picture everything on a buffet table as at least 100 calories for every three bites. It adds up fast.
6. Drink lots of water or club soda to keep you hydrated and full.
7. Don't hesitate to leave food on your plate. If it isn't awesomely delicious, don't finish it.

Cutting Calories Daily

CALORIES ADD UP FAST

You can find unlimited ways to reduce calories and fat from your food. From buttering your toast to preparing a gourmet meal, you can use creative techniques to create delicious and healthier alternatives. You can find many excellent light-cooking magazines or cookbooks at any local bookstore. Never forget that every calorie counts. If you creatively save 200 calories each day, you could be 20 pounds lighter in a year!

CONCENTRATED CALORIES

Some foods we need to eat sparingly because they are so high in calories, such as cheese, olives, avocados, and nuts. While they are satisfying and healthful in small amounts, we can very easily eat too much. Flavor your foods with these rich treats, but try not to make them a substantial part of your meal or snack. I do recommend nuts as snacks since they are such a great source of protein, fiber, and healthy fat—BUT measure out servings of one ounce and stop at that!

I hardly need to say that other high-calorie "fun foods" like candy, cookies, and pastries add up fast. No foods are "forbidden," yet these rich and satisfying treats can make a big dent in your calorie bank account. I encourage you to get tuned in to how much fat and how many calories are really in that mud pie and chocolate cheesecake they serve at your favorite restaurant. The truth alone will scare you into sharing your dessert and even leaving a few bites on the plate.

Healthy Eating and Cooking Ideas

When you go on a traditional weight loss diet, you are given a list of foods you can and cannot eat and often the amount that is acceptable. That's great if you follow it to a T, because you have no room to fail. But even if the diet works, you still have to figure out how to eat in the real world and *keep the weight off*. The reason I am so opposed to structured eating plans is because we are all so different. Making a lifestyle change may be a little more work up front and take a little longer for you to get in the "groove," but for those who are willing to do the work, the results will be long lasting.

That is why I encourage you to take some time to think about your eating challenges. Identifying when and where you have your greatest struggles is helpful. For many people it is toward the end of the day. But you may start the day off wrong with too much coffee, with simple carbohydrates, or with no breakfast at all. Whatever your issues, identify them and create a strategy for addressing them.

The lists below may help you deal with some of your key areas. Take a highlighter and mark the suggestions that appeal to you. Then take action and implement them.

Calorie-Busting at Breakfast

1. Eat your toast with jam and no butter or margarine.
2. On those rare occasions that you *do* have pancakes, waffles, or French toast, avoid using butter and just top them with reduced sugar syrup or jam. Pancakes are generally the lowest-calorie choice. Make your own in a nonstick pan.
3. Scramble 1 egg yolk and 2 egg whites and save 120 calories!
4. Make an omelet with egg whites or egg substitutes and add lots of your favorite chopped vegetables for flavor and fiber.
5. Read the labels on all bread, bagel, and muffin packages to find the healthiest, lowest-calorie, highest-fiber choice. Oroweat makes some of the best.

Calorie-Busting Snacks

1. Many tasty popcorn choices can be low calorie. Be sure to read the portion size accurately.
2. Try frozen grapes or blueberries for a healthy snack.
3. Can't resist your occasional potato chip? Try Baked Lays—they're wonderful. Or buy a single one-ounce bag of your very favorite kind, sit down, and slowly eat all 150 calories!
4. Mix ½ ounce of nuts (90 calories) with half of a sliced apple. You'll be satisfied and fibered up!
5. Hard candy or mints are low in calories and satisfy the sweet tooth. They also take about three or four minutes to eat.
6. Graham crackers with a thin layer of peanut butter and warm herbal tea satisfy sweet cravings with less sugar and fat.
7. Avoid the guacamole and stick with low-calorie salsa. If you can't resist the avocado, mix it with generous amounts of salsa and fresh tomatoes. And use carrots or celery for dipping between the *one ounce* of chips you've pre-measured!
8. Use cheese as a condiment; leave it off your sandwiches and burgers, cut the amount in recipes in half, and avoid snacking on this dangerously high fat morsel.

9. High-fat chips and buttery crackers can pile on calories quickly. Always pre-measure (or mentally calculate the amount) before you eat. If you can't be satisfied with one ounce, avoid them.

Calorie-Busting When Eating Out

1. Order one Caesar salad and one plain mixed salad and toss them together to lower the calories and fat. Or just ask the waiter to cut the dressing in half before they toss your salad.
2. Bypass fatty salad bar extras such as sunflower seeds, high-fat croutons, chow mein noodles, and bacon bits. All those extras could add several hundred calories to your meal!
3. Carry your own reduced fat salad dressings. Too many tasty and healthy dressings are now available to ever settle for high-fat choices.
4. Order an appetizer as an entrée at restaurants that serve huge portions. Light soup or salad and a small appetizer provides plenty of calories.
5. Flank steak, London broil, and filet mignon are lower fat steak choices. Ask for the smallest option and eat about four ounces. Take the rest home.
6. Order pizza with a thin crust, ⅓ less cheese (or light cheese), and lots of veggies. Save about 100 to 150 calories per slice.
7. Always select "red" sauce versus "white" with your pasta. White sauce is usually high in cream, which means fat! Don't hesitate to order your sauce on the side. You can also ask them to prepare it with less oil.
8. Order a baked potato with the condiments on the side instead of french fries. New potatoes taste great and require less butter since they are moister than bakers.
9. Drain oily sauce from Chinese meals by lifting the food from the serving dish onto your plate with chopsticks or a fork.
10. Research all your regular fast food restaurants online and pull up their nutritional information. Determine what the healthiest choices are and be ready to order those next time you drive through. (Go to a search engine and just put in the name of the restaurant,

and you will almost always get a list that will include the restaurant's website with all the information you need. Be prepared to be shocked if you've never researched the calorie content of your favorite fast foods!)

Healthy Cooking Tips

1. Brown ground turkey or lean beef in a nonstick pan; then drain with hot water in a colander to remove excess fat.
2. Precook your baked potatoes in the microwave for 5 to 8 minutes and then place in a 500-degree oven for about 10 minutes to make them fluffy. Don't forget to eat the skin!
3. Buy low-fat spaghetti sauces and add fresh onion, mushrooms, peppers, and zucchini to increase the fiber and give it a homemade taste.
4. Make your own low-fat burritos. Buy low-fat tortillas, canned black beans, and fresh cilantro and tomatoes, and you've got a great source of protein and fiber.
5. Buy small packages of fresh herbs to add to many recipes for extra flavor. Food should never be bland—experiment!
6. Buy boneless, skinless chicken tenders and cook enough for a whole week. Throw them in salads, soups, pita bread, burritos, stir-fry, or whatever!
7. Try a variety of low- or nonfat marinades that are on the market to enhance any chicken, turkey, or beef dish.
8. Use grains like couscous, kashi, or brown rice as a base for many different meals such as:
   - chili with cornbread
   - petite peas and diced chicken tenders
   - stir-fried veggies
   - London broil and grilled peppers, onions, and sweet potatoes
9. Bake a sweet potato and mix in a small amount of light butter and 2 teaspoons of brown sugar. It's satisfying and packed with antioxidants and lots of fiber.

10. Buy fresh pastas and toss with a tablespoon of olive oil and one tablespoon of seasoned feta cheese crumbled very small. Add fresh herbs.
11. Create your own lower fat salad dressing by mixing a flavored vinegar with your favorite higher fat dressing.
12. Sauté foods in chicken or vegetable broth, tomato juice, or wine for lots of flavor and low calories!
13. Keep olive oil in a spray bottle to lightly coat cookware.
14. Make your own taco shells by hanging soft tortillas directly over the racks in your oven and baking at 400 degrees until crisp.
15. Refrigerate homemade soups overnight. Skim off the fat on top in the morning and save tons of calories!
16. Cook rice, couscous, and other grains in chicken broth and NO butter. It tastes great!
17. Thicken cream sauces with 1-percent milk and cornstarch instead of butter and flour.
18. Trim visible fat from meat and remove the skin from all poultry.
19. Use cocktail sauce or lemon juice instead of tartar sauce on fish.
20. Reduce the amount of meat or poultry in your fajitas, casseroles, or other dishes and increase the vegetables, rice, or beans.
21. Make your own eggplant or vegetable lasagna with low fat or less cheese.
22. Choose barbequed chicken instead of pork or beef. Remove the skin before baking your own.

Lighter Choices

1. Switch from canned baked beans made with pork to vegetarian varieties.
2. Never eat high-fat ice cream. Too many excellent low-fat and non-fat alternatives are available. You'll potentially save hundreds of calories.
3. Check out the wide variety of dehydrated soups. Many are low in fat and very high in fiber. They are also easy to take to work. (Do watch for high sodium content and use in moderation those that are high.)

4. Croissants contain about 300 calories from fat. They're not worth it! Stick with your favorite fresh bread.

5. Use less low-fat mayonnaise in tuna or chicken salad by adding a little low-fat dressing such as rice vinegar.

6 Opt for white-meat poultry instead of dark meat. Never eat the skin.

7 Artichokes with low-fat mayonnaise or low-calorie dips are nutritious and delicious. Try nonfat plain yogurt for your dip recipes also.

8 All tortillas are not equal. Read the labels and buy the smaller, lower-fat, and no-lard selections.

9. Avoid buying highly processed and fatty luncheon meats like bologna, hotdogs, and salami. Instead eat lean chicken and turkey.

10. Eat a turkey sandwich instead of chicken salad (save 200 to 300 calories).

11. Choose albacore tuna packed in water instead of oil. (You'll get your omega-3 fatty acids too!)

12. Eggnog-flavored coffee creamer has a lot fewer calories than eggnog. Make a fresh cup of coffee with special flavor for dessert.

13. Reduce the amount of butter, mayonnaise, and other spreads on your breads, rolls, etc. The spread should totally blend into the surface of your food. Scrape off any excess with your knife before you take the first bite. You could save hundreds of calories per week changing this one habit and be 10–20 pounds leaner in a year!

14. Choose rolls instead of high-fat biscuits.

15. Leave the cheese off your sandwich and add tomatoes, cucumbers, or pickles.

16. Learn how to read labels correctly for fat and calorie content. Try to select snacks and desserts that are no more than 30 percent fat. Warning: check out the serving size—it's often very small.

17. Love cheese? Select Parmesan or low-fat mozzarella. Buy sharper cheeses for more flavor and use less.

18. Avoid regular mayonnaise, especially if you are mixing it with something. Cut low-fat mayonnaise with dijon mustard to decrease the calories and increase the flavor.

Calorie-Busting Desserts

1. Sprinkle nuts on top of homemade desserts as a "flavoring" instead of mixing in the batter where the full flavor and texture may get lost.
2. Order one dessert for everyone at your table and share!
3. Substitute applesauce for some of the oil in your favorite recipes. Replace the oil with the same amount of applesauce.
4. Look for recipes that use cocoa powder (which has no fat) in place of chocolate.
5. Order low-fat, decaf lattes, cappuccinos, and other low-calorie specialty drinks instead of dessert.
6. Sip low-calorie hot cocoa to satisfy a chocolate craving.
7. Angel food cake can be dressed up in many ways for a non-fat dessert. Try making a chocolate angel food cake—yum!
8. Lower-fat cookies include biscotti, vanilla-filled wafers, Oreos, and meringues. Read the labels.
9. Low-fat frozen yogurt with a special sauce or flavor is a wonderful treat. Try fruit sorbet with berries.
10. Once a week, go ahead and simply indulge in your favorite dessert, but eat only a third or a half of your usual portion.

Healthy Eating

Despite my aversion to creating eating plans, I do understand that many of you would like some ideas for getting enough protein, fiber, and other key nutrients in your diet. I've included some favorite meal and snack choices that I eat on a regular basis. In some cases, I've included specific brands.

At the very end of this chapter, I've also added nine recipes that have been enjoyed by many friends or clients. You can find an abundance of healthy cookbooks on the market today. They include excellent recipes, and you can also learn creative ways to cut calories in some of your favorite recipes by following some of their substitution principles.

Protein/Fiber Breakfast Choices

Protein shake	400 calories / 16g protein / 11g fiber
Hard-boiled egg	1 large / 75 calories / 7g protein
Egg Beaters	¼ cup / 100 calories / 7g protein
Custard	150 calories / 12g protein
Oat bran cereal (cooked)	⅓ cup uncooked / 140 calories / 8g protein / 7g fiber
Bob's Red Mill Cereal	¼ cup dry / 140 calories / 6g protein / 5g fiber (order online at www.bobsredmill.com)
Bran flakes	1 cup / 110 calories / 8g protein / 4–6g fiber
Peanut butter	1 Tbsp / 100 calories / 4.5g protein
Oroweat Light Whole Wheat Bread	2 slices / 80 calories / 7g fiber
1% milk	1 cup / 110 calories / 10g protein
Vanilla low-fat yogurt	½ cup / 95 calories / 6g protein

Note: Increase fiber by adding fresh fruit, berries, or small amounts of nuts or flaxseeds to hot cereals or whole grain pancakes. Avoid juices and eat the whole fruit instead. Add non-flavored protein powder to hot cereals if you want to increase the protein without preparing eggs or a meat. Remember that you ideally want to get a minimum of 15 grams of protein with breakfast.

Protein/Fiber Lunch and Dinner Choices

Fresh or canned salmon	2 ounces / 80 calories / 12g protein
Low-fat burrito	6 ounces / 260 calories / 13g protein / 7g fiber
Cattle Drive Chicken Chili	1 cup / 190 calories / 17g protein / 1g fiber
Progresso Beef Barley Soup	1 cup / 110 calories / 8g protein / 3g fiber
Teriyaki Chicken Bowl	354g / 460 calories / 20g protein / 3g fiber
Cottage cheese	½ cup / 14g protein
Chicken breast (skinless)	4 ounces / 190 calories / 42g protein / 22 calories from fat
Lots of veggies	about 3–4 grams of fiber per serving

Note: Add pinto, black, white, or kidney beans to salads, soups, and casseroles for an excellent source of fiber and additional protein. Add a wide variety of chopped veggies to soups and sauces as well for increased flavor and nutritional value.

Healthy Snack Choices

Balance Bar	1 bar / 210 calories / 15g protein
Most nuts	1 ounce / 160 calories / 6g protein / 3g fiber
Olives	8 olives / 50 calories
Whole wheat crackers	3 crackers / 110 calories / 2g protein / 1g fiber
Most fruits	100 to 150 calories each / 3g fiber
Baby carrots	3 ounces / 40 calories / 3g fiber

Eating with Danna in the Real World

People ask me all the time how I eat on a day-to-day basis. Well, how I eat may not be what you would enjoy. However, just for kicks, here's an example of how I ate the day after Thanksgiving. You'll note that I ate just under 2,000 calories, which I happen to know is exactly how many I burned that day because I went for a 400-calorie walk (according to my Caltrac activity monitor). You can see how easy it is to eat that many calories without going overboard. You can also see in my second example that with some very minor modifications, I could easily decrease that by 600 calories. I hope this example will help you realize how small choices make a big difference day after day—not just the day after Thanksgiving.

THE DAY AFTER THANKSGIVING: 1,985 CALORIES

Breakfast
½ cup Egg Beaters with ½ ounce of cheddar cheese
1 piece "Orowheat Light" brand toast, lightly buttered
Coffee with 1 tablespoon of cream
400 calories / 14g protein / 4g fiber

Snack
Green tea
Balance Bar
200 calories / 15g protein

Lunch
3 ounces turkey with ¼ cup cranberry sauce
3 ounces baby carrots
½ cup of stuffing (just because it tastes great)
½ cup green bean casserole
450 calories / 18g protein / 6g fiber

Snack
1 ounce of almonds
1 apple
260 calories / 6g protein / 6g fiber

Dinner
2 cups turkey vegetable and noodle soup
1 sourdough roll
Green salad with balsamic vinegar and olive oil
450 calories / 25g protein / 6g fiber

Dessert
Decaf coffee with one tablespoon cream
½ piece homemade apple/raspberry pie (left ½ of crust)
225 calories

Total: 1,985 calories / 78g protein / 22g fiber

MODIFIED DAY AFTER THANKSGIVING: 1,425 CALORIES

Breakfast
½ cup Egg Beaters
1 piece Oroweat toast, lightly buttered
½ banana
Coffee with cream
395 calories / 14g protein / 6g fiber

Snack
Green tea
½ Balance Bar
100 calories / 7.5g protein

Lunch
3 ounces turkey with ¼ cup cranberry sauce
3 ounces baby carrots
½ cup green bean casserole
Sliced apple

450 calories / 18g protein / 9g fiber

Snack
½ ounce of almonds
80 calories / 3g protein / 3g fiber

Dinner
2 cups turkey vegetable and noodle soup
Green salad with balsamic vinegar and olive oil
300 calories / 25g protein / 6g fiber

Dessert:
Decaf coffee with cream
2 Hershey's Kisses
100 calories

Total: 1,425 calories / 67.5g protein / 24g fiber
Resource: www.TheCalorieCounter.com

Personal Reflection

Answer the following questions on your own or with your group:

1. As you reviewed all the healthy eating and cooking ideas, what were the top three ideas you liked?

2. What are your greatest weaknesses in how you shop, eat, or cook?

3. What will you do to improve in these areas?

4. Are you a procrastinator? Yes or no, *now* is a great time to take action. Begin to create your shopping list today. Keep adding to it over the next day, and then schedule a time to go shopping when you are not in a hurry, taking extra care to read labels and look for healthier food choices.

Build a Strong Spiritual Foundation

Meditate on the following Scripture and answer the corresponding questions:

Search me, O God, and know my heart; try me and know my anxious thoughts; and see if there be any hurtful way in me, and lead me in the everlasting way.

Psalm 139:23–24

1. Of course, the psalmist knew that God knew his heart through and through. But his desire was for God to reflect it back to him and to lead him down the right path. This is a great example of surrender. How can you surrender your struggles more fully to the Lord?

2. What are your anxious thoughts with respect to your body or lifestyle?

3. Since God told us in Philippians 4:6 to "be anxious for nothing," how do we apply this in our lives in a practical way?

4. Many people are living under great stress and anxiety, which contributes to overeating and many health and relational issues. Spend time this week evaluating and praying about the stress and/or anxiety in your life.

Nourish Your Spirit

Life-changing spiritual victory requires daily nourishment. Continue to nourish your spirit daily in four ways:

1. Pray as if it is the air you breathe.

This week make a practice of saying a prayer before putting anything into your mouth. When you ask God to bless the food, also ask him to convict you if you are making poor choices or eating too much.

2. Nourish your soul and spirit with God's Word daily.

Are you in the Word daily? If yes, great! If not, take at least five minutes each day to nourish yourself with the most important nutrient available—God's truth.

3. Digest its truths through meditation.

Meditate on our verses, Psalm 139:23–34, for this week and ask the Lord to reveal the areas of your heart and mind that need renewal. Let him lead you in the everlasting way that brings great peace. Do a word search on the word "peace" in the New Testament and see what you learn about dealing with stress and anxiety.

4. Practice the presence of God.

How have you been doing with becoming aware of God's continual presence in your life? How is this impacting your life? Make a lifetime commitment to grow in this exercise. For greater inspiration in this area, read the story of Brother Lawrence called *Practicing the Presence of God* or A. W. Tozer's book *The Pursuit of God*.

Prayer for Week Seven

Dear Lord, I desire to put the truths I learn from your Word and from this program into practice. Help me to have wisdom when I shop, cook, and eat out. I pray that your Spirit will prompt me with a conviction of how each choice makes a difference and bring to mind the ideas I have learned. I also ask that you help me to manage my time in a way that puts my health as a priority. Teach me and transform me in your perfect timing. In Jesus's name, Amen.

Suggested Reading for Week Seven

Practicing the Presence of God by Brother Lawrence

The Pursuit of God by A. W. Tozer

Healthy cookbooks

Favorite Recipes

Resource: LivingCookbook.com

A wonderful computer program is available from www.livingcook book.com. You can enter any recipe and it will kick out a complete nutrition label and compile a cookbook, shopping list, and more for you. So if you're wondering about the nutritional value of all those yummy family recipes, here's an easy way to find out. You can download it for a free trial of twenty-five uses or purchase it for $30.00.

Danna's Healthy Custard

2 cups of 1-percent low-fat milk
3 lightly beaten eggs (or egg substitute equivalent)
¼ cup sugar
¼ teaspoon salt
½ teaspoon vanilla

Scald milk in a saucepan. Remove from heat and slowly stir in eggs. Then stir in salt, sugar, and vanilla. Pour into 6 custard cups and sprinkle with nutmeg or cinnamon. Bake in a pan of hot water at 325 degrees for 30 to 40 minutes.

Potato and Bell Pepper Frittata

1 Tbsp olive oil
8 oz. red potatoes, thinly sliced
½ cup sliced red onion
½ of a red bell pepper, thinly sliced
½ of a yellow bell pepper, thinly
  sliced
½ cup broccoli, chopped

2 tsp fresh chopped sage or dried
  rubbed sage
1 tsp salt
½ tsp freshly ground pepper
8 eggs
2 cups plus ¼ cup shredded Parmesan
  cheese

1. Preheat oven to 350. Heat olive oil in a 12-inch nonstick ovenproof skillet over medium heat. Add potatoes, onion, bell peppers, and broccoli; cover and cook, stirring occasionally, until vegetables are tender, about 10 minutes. Stir in 1 teaspoon of the sage, ½ teaspoon of the salt, and ¼ teaspoon of the pepper.

2. Whisk together the eggs, 2 cups of the cheese, and the remaining sage, salt, and pepper; pour over vegetables in skillet and cook until edges of eggs just begin to set, about 3 minutes.

3. Sprinkle top with the remaining cheese and bake until center is set, about 8 minutes. Invert onto a serving plate. Makes 4 servings.

Nutritional Analysis: 435 calories, 27g fat, 33g protein, 14g carbohydrates.

Salmon with Maple Syrup and Toasted Almonds

Six 6-ounce salmon fillets
Cooking spray
¼ cup packed brown sugar
¼ cup maple syrup

3 Tbsp low-sodium soy sauce
1 Tbsp Dijon mustard
¼ tsp black pepper
4 tsp sliced almonds, toasted

Preheat oven to 425. Place fillets in a 9- by 13-inch baking dish coated with cooking spray. Combine sugar, syrup, soy sauce, mustard, and black pepper; pour sugar mixture over fillets. Cover with foil; bake at 425 for 10 minutes. Remove foil; sprinkle the fillets with almonds. Bake an additional 10 minutes or until fish flakes easily when tested with a fork. Serve with sugar mixture. Yields 6 servings.

Nutritional Analysis: 373 calories, 12.78g total fat (2.56 saturated fat), 418mg sodium, 799mg potassium, 43g protein.

Couscous, Black Bean, and Feta Salad

Easy, delicious, and nutritious! A great potluck dish too.

1 can (15 oz.) black beans, rinsed and
  drained
1½ cups chopped tomatoes
1½ cups (or 1 box) plain couscous, cooked
1 pkg (4 oz.) crumbled feta cheese
2 Tbsp chopped fresh cilantro or parsley

½ cup chopped celery
½ cup chopped green onions
½ cup fat-free Italian dressing

Mix all ingredients and refrigerate. Makes 5 servings.

Nutritional Analysis: 222 calories, 5.6g total fat (3.56 saturated fat), 683mg sodium, 468mg potassium, 7.45g fiber, 4.65g sugar, 12g protein.

Seven-Vegetable Salad

A beautiful, crisp, and flavorful salad!

1 cup cut fresh green beans
1 cup fresh sugar snap peas
1 cup sliced yellow summer squash
1 cup sliced zucchini
½ cup julienne onion

2 small tomatoes, seeded and chopped
1 cup coarsely grated carrots
⅔ cup low-fat Italian salad dressing
4 tsp minced chives
2 tsp dried basil

In a saucepan, bring 2 inches of water to a boil. Add beans, peas, yellow squash, zucchini, and onion. Reduce heat; cover and simmer for 2–3 minutes or until vegetables are crisp-tender. Drain; rinse with cold water and pat dry. Place vegetables in a bowl; add the remaining ingredients. Gently stir to coat. Refrigerate until serving. Yields 12 servings.

Nutritional Analysis: ½ cup equals 47 calories, 2g fat, 132mg sodium, 6g carbohydrates, 2g fiber, 1g protein.

Chicken Parmigiana

½ cup dry bread crumbs
3 Tbsp grated Parmesan cheese
¾ tsp Italian seasoning
½ tsp garlic powder
½ tsp salt

¼ cup egg substitute
4 boneless, skinless chicken breast halves
1 jar (26 oz.) meatless spaghetti sauce
¾ cup shredded part-skim mozzarella
¼ cup shredded Parmesan

In a shallow bowl, combine the bread crumbs, grated Parmesan, Italian seasoning, garlic powder, and salt. In another bowl, beat egg substitute. Dip chicken in egg substitute, then roll in crumbs. Place in a 9- by 13- by 2-inch baking dish coated with nonstick cooking spray. Bake uncovered at 375 degrees for 10 minutes. Turn chicken; bake for 10 minutes. Pour spaghetti sauce over chicken; bake for 5 minutes. Sprinkle with cheeses; bake 10 minutes longer or until chicken juices run clear. Yields 4 servings.

Nutritional Analysis: 412 calories, 15g fat (5g saturated), 88mg cholesterol, 1420mg sodium, 32g carbohydrate, 5g fiber, 37g protein.

Vegetable Quiche Cups to Go

¾ cup to 1 cup egg substitute (about 4 eggs)
¾ cup shredded reduced-fat cheese
¼ cup diced onion
¼ cup diced green pepper
¼ cup diced celery
1 pkg. frozen chopped spinach
salt, pepper, and hot sauce (3–6 drops) to taste
12 foil cupcake liners

Preheat oven to 350 degrees. Place foil cupcake liners in muffin pan. Spray nonstick cooking spray into the cupcake liners. Microwave the frozen spinach for 2½ minutes on high. Squeeze all the excess liquid from the spinach. In a mixing bowl combine spinach, onion, celery, egg substitute, cheese, salt, and pepper to taste. Add hot sauce if desired. Mix well. Spoon mixture evenly into the 12 cupcake liners. Bake in the oven about 20 minutes or until knife inserted in center comes out clean. Can be frozen and reheated in the microwave (without foil liners). A good breakfast or lunch alternative.

Nutritional Analysis: 2 quiches equals 77 calories, 9g protein, 3g carbohydrates, 2g fiber.

Week Eight:
The Click Factor

In This Section:

What's a "Click Factor"?

Writing Your Own Powerful Self-Talk

What's a "Click Factor"?

Teaching people how to make lasting lifestyle changes can be a frustrating venture. No matter how much knowledge you give, how many great ideas you provide, or how inspiring your enthusiasm or personal testimony, you have no control over what the recipients will ultimately do. I have finally resolved that my job is to impart truth. In the end, I must leave the results up to you and God.

In the revised edition of *Scale Down*, I added some teaching on the subject of what I've come to call the "click factor." The click factor is the experience, attitude, or perspective that will motivate you sufficiently and sustain you indefinitely in your quest for a leaner and healthier body. If you find it, you've most likely discovered *your key* to permanent victory. I think that this concept is important enough to repeat in this workbook. I encourage you to review the concept and then actually go on a journey to discover your key if you have not already.

I get email from all over the country from both men and women who are actually "clicking" as they read *Scale Down* and begin implementing the principles. When I get the opportunity to speak personally with someone, I always want to know what "clicked" for them. I have two examples that I hope will inspire you to find your "click factor."

Small Steps Add Up

When *Scale Down* was first released in March 2003, I had the privilege of being interviewed on one of the most popular and most widely broadcast Christian radio talk shows in the country, *Midday Connection*. The interviewer, Anita Lustrea, works for Moody Broadcasting and was a wonderfully enthusiastic host. She was excited about the principles I taught, asked great questions, and juggled an hour's worth of calls from her listeners as I answered questions on every aspect of lifestyle change. The really cool thing was that six months later, when she asked me back for another interview, she revealed on air that she had lost 35 pounds since reading *Scale Down*. Now, almost three years later, she has lost a total of 50 pounds and kept it off. When asked what "clicked" for her, Anita said that she finally realized that *little things really did add up* when she practiced them *consistently*. As she started eating more protein and fiber, her energy increased and she began to move more. One day at a time, each little change slowly brought more visible rewards, and she thought, *I can do this for a lifetime*!

Worn-Out Tapes

In late 2004 I received a call from a client who had taken my eight-week program about three years earlier. In her message she said that she had lost 100 pounds, had completely worn out her self-talk tapes (now in CD format), and needed a new set for continued encouragement. For Kathleen the "click factor" was learning the power of transforming her mind with healthy thinking about food and her body. Even more exciting was the fact that she did not even know Christ as her Savior when she first took the program . . . but she does now! As of this writing,

Kathleen has become an important part of our *Scale Down* team and is helping us facilitate classes in San Diego.

In addition to using the healthy self-talk tapes, Kathleen did a great job identifying her lies and writing new, positive self-talk very specific to her life. She also found great benefit in recording some of her own messages in her own voice. That is why I asked her to contribute to this week's study by sharing how she did this. I have a very strong sense that this is probably the single most important "click factor" for most people: reprogramming your self-talk.

Trigger Talk—Just Do It!

After you go through the exercise below individually or with your group, please do yourself a *huge* favor and begin practicing your "trigger talk" as discussed in the section "You Are What You Think" in week three. The time you take to write or record new messages will be without value if you don't consistently tell yourself those truths day after day, week after week, month after month. If you want to experience victory like Anita and Kathleen, take some consistent small steps and speak truth daily into your own mind. Then call me so I can celebrate with you!

Writing Your Own Powerful Self-Talk

Kathleen defines healthy self-talk in this way: *"Statements of truth that I want to believe, said as if I already believe them."* As you've already learned, *healthy* self-talk is first and foremost about telling yourself truth. But it's not truth as you are living it but rather truth of the potential and possibility of what you can do and be *if and when* you surrender to God's principles and purpose for your life. Here are some of Kathleen's suggestions for writing your own healthy, truth-based self-talk.

Guidelines for Writing Your Own Self-Talk

1. Keep it positive. Avoid using negative words like *no, never*, or *can't*.

2. Keep it in the present. Avoid using words like *will*, *should*, or *going to*. Instead use phrases like *I am* or *I have*.

3. Make it memorable. Unless you are recording a self-talk cassette to listen to, keep your statements simple and easy to recall and repeat (especially in times of temptation). For recordings, studies have shown that people actually learn faster when studying while listening to baroque music. Try playing Mozart or Beethoven in the background.

4. Remember, the most dominant thought wins. You will believe what you tell yourself most often, so personalize a few self-talk messages and make them part of your daily life. Be sure to include self-talk to balance all three areas of your life: physical, mental, and spiritual.

5. Go back to your four evaluations and notice how most statements are worded positively. Circle the ones you rated lowest and use some of those statements for your personal self-talk.

6. Find two or three Scripture verses that speak directly to your personal challenges. Memorize them and use them when you feel tempted, defeated, or low.

Positive Self-Talk Examples

Instead of:	Change to:
I will not eat junk food.	I choose to eat healthy food and love it.
I should take better care of myself.	I deserve good health and take good care of myself.
I will lose 20 pounds.	I am eating and exercising for maximum health.

Self-Talk Examples for Each Dimension

Physical: I enjoy exercise and love the way it makes me feel!

Mental: I am strong and Christ-confident with a positive life and perspective.

Spiritual: I am an obedient and faithful child of God. I know I can do all things through Christ who strengthens me.

Personal Reflection

Answer the following questions on your own or with your group:

1. How are you doing? Now that you have been on your journey for a while, take time to revisit how you are "balancing the dimensions of your life." On a scale from 1 to 10 (with 10 being the best), how do you rate yourself in the following areas?

   - My physical health and wellness: _____
   - My thoughts, life perspective, attitudes about life: _____
   - My emotions, feelings about myself and others: _____
   - My behavior such as habits, lifestyle, work, and stress: _____
   - My spiritual dimension, time with God, life purpose: _____

2. What about your "one thing"? Once again, what is the "one thing" in each area that will make the biggest difference in experiencing victory in that dimension? Pray for wisdom to know what that is and the appropriate and God-honoring action to take. Then write it down next to each area below:

   - My physical health and wellness "one thing":
   _____
   - My thoughts, life perspective, attitudes about life "one thing":
   _____
   - My emotions, feelings about myself and others "one thing":
   _____
   - My behavior such as habits, lifestyle, work, and stress "one thing": _____
   - My spiritual dimension, time with God, life purpose "one thing": _____

3. Take action: paper, prayer, and practice! Spend some time this week deciding how you are going to weave these actions into your life. This is a very important exercise that should take considerable prayer, reflection, and planning.

Build a Strong Spiritual Foundation

Meditate on this Scripture and answer the corresponding questions:

And He said to him, "You shall love the Lord Your God with all your heart, and with all your soul, and with all your mind."

Matthew 22:37

1. How do you develop an all-consuming love for God?

2. How does that kind of love change your life?

3. What can you do every day to deepen your love for God?

4. What is stopping you from doing that every day?

5. What will you do specifically this week to make your relationship with God the single most important thing in your life?

Nourish Your Spirit

Life-changing spiritual victory requires daily nourishment. Nourish your spirit daily in four ways:

1. Pray as if it is the air you breathe.

Matthew 22:37 is the core of all things important. When we experience this kind of love for God, our thoughts, feelings, and behaviors will follow. Pray daily that God will impart to you the ability to love him first and foremost.

2. Nourish your soul and spirit with God's Word daily.

To know and love God, we must know and love his Word, since that is how he communicates with us. Remind yourself that his love letter is waiting to be read and reread so you will discover and experience the depth and breadth of his love which is beyond comprehension.

3. Digest its truths through meditation.

Memorize our verse this week and use it in your "trigger time" for the next several weeks. This will help you make the next step (practicing the presence of God) a daily reality in your life.

4. Practice the presence of God.

Go back through the last seven weeks' studies and list all the ideas for practicing God's presence. Write down two or three which are most helpful to you and *do them*! He is here with you right now—and will be forever. Wouldn't it be incredible if that reality was always in the forefront of our thoughts?

Prayer for Week Eight

Heavenly Father, thank you for the journey we have been on together. I know that it has only just begun and that I need your strength and guidance to stay on the path of healthy thinking and living. Please empower me with your Spirit and give me the wisdom and self-discipline that comes only from you to stay the course. I praise you that you have made all things new and that I will someday know ultimate perfection. I love you, Lord. Amen.

Week Nine (Optional):
A Personality-Powered Lifestyle

In This Section:

Personality Blueprints

Personality Profile

Personality Scoring Sheet

Lifestyle Guides for the Four Personalities

In order to effectively implement change in your life, you must be aware of all the factors that will enhance or inhibit change. That is why I put so much emphasis on the mental dimension and surrender to God. Another area critical to your success is an understanding of your personal temperament.

Personality Blueprints

We are all designed with a specific personality blueprint. We can see clearly as we observe people that we don't all react the same way to a given situation. Since the Greek physician Hippocrates, scholars have observed four distinct personalities. Perhaps you have had an opportunity to take a personality profile. No matter what names the personalities are given, experts agree on four basic profiles. You are usually a combination of two. As a certified personality trainer, I refer to them as follows:

- the popular Sanguine who loves to have fun
- the powerful Choleric who wants control
- the perfect Melancholy who needs perfection
- the peaceful Phlegmatic who wants peace at all costs

In my experience, the most desperate and frustrated clients have been the ones trying to make changes according to someone else's formula or standard which is completely contrary to their personality.

To understand this better, let's take an intimate look into the lives of four individuals with four distinctly different personalities. Perhaps one or more will sound uncomfortably familiar. Don't let their stories get you too depressed. You will read constructive and appropriate suggestions for each personality at the end. A personality profile analysis and recommendations for your lifestyle according to your personality type follows this. You will learn how each unique temperament can be influenced in both positive and negative ways. By identifying your own personality blueprint, you will be able to more effectively design a lifestyle plan that can work specifically for you!

The Sanguine Solution: Sharon, a Yo-yo Dieter, Focused on Quick Fixes and Diet Aids

"Oh my gosh! It's too small; my favorite dress is too small! What happened?" Sharon squealed as she stood gawking in the full-length mirror. Her husband, Dan, came running, thinking something was terribly wrong, only to find Sharon huffing and puffing around the bedroom with seemingly dozens of outfits thrown onto the bed. "Sharon, we have to leave for the party in ten minutes! What are you doing?" Dan questioned, the irritation seeping into his voice. Frustrated, Sharon responded, "I'm trying to find something to wear! Everything is too tight; I don't know what's happened."

Dan rolled his eyes out of Sharon's view. This had happened many times before. Sharon had been a yo-yo dieter for years. She rotated in a circle of size 6, 8, 10, and back to 6 again in about three-year cycles. He had figured years ago that it was how she justified doing so much shopping. Her frequent excuse was, "Nothing fits!"

A bigger concern than simply the budget and Sharon's obvious current frustration was coming to the surface. Dan had noticed that she seemed more and more focused on quick fixes and diet aids.

In the past four years, they had acquired a stationary bike, a stair-stepper, and many other weights and gadgets. When she got bored with these after two or three weeks, she had convinced Dan that a gym membership was the answer. Unfortunately, Sharon found the people at the gym too serious. They tried to put her on a program of aerobics and weight training, but she just wasn't having fun.

In addition, Sharon had filled their cupboards with every vitamin and pill imaginable, each label declaring some new "fat-burning formula." Fat-free frozen treats overflowed in the freezer and low-fat or no-fat sweets were everywhere. With all this low-fat eating, the exercise equipment, and the gym membership, why was Sharon having such difficulty? More important, why had she lost her normally energetic and vivacious spirit?

The popular Sanguine Sharon had always been full of life and optimism. Dan had watched her sacrifice nutrition for taste and good common sense for results. She seemed much more concerned with how she looked than with how she felt.

His concerns increased considerably over the next several months. Almost miraculously, Sharon seemed to be melting off her most recent weight gain and was back in her favorite size 6 dress within ten weeks. At first she seemed to be her old energetic self, full of life and happiness. But the more she lost, the more irritable and forgetful she became. It reached its peak one Wednesday when their eight-year-old son, Josh, called Dan at the office, sobbing, "Dad, I've been standing outside school for an hour in the rain. I think Mom forgot to pick me up!"

Dan confronted Sharon with his concerns, and she flew off the handle, claiming her forgetfulness was due to lack of sleep. "What are you taking, anyway, Sharon? This can't be good for you," Dan pressed.

"Dan, my doctor prescribed it; it's totally safe. It's the latest, most effective medication. He's monitoring me closely. I'm just fine. And besides, I look better than when I was in my twenties!"

"Actually, the last few weeks, you look too thin," he retorted. "What doctor in his right mind would continue giving diet pills to someone who doesn't need to lose weight?"

"That's it, Dan!" Sharon hollered back. "You just don't want me to look this good, do you?"

The fight escalated, and Sharon's irritability increased. The symptoms of nervousness and forgetfulness became harder to deny over the next few weeks. She slept through her alarm three days in a row and left Josh waiting thirty minutes one more afternoon before admitting it was time to put away the pills. Sadly, the weight began to come back, more quickly than before. Five months later and almost back in her size 10 jeans, she saw the advertisement in her local paper and knew she had to go . . .

The Choleric "Complex": Frank, Stressed-Out "Type A" Business Executive

Frank could feel the tension rising up his neck as he slammed down the receiver and pushed the intercom button on his phone. "Martha! Send Mr. Gibson the Donnelly proposal, yesterday! What in the #*!& is wrong with this company? The mailroom loses everything. And we may end up losing our largest account!"

"No problem, Frank. Just relax. I'll express mail it. He'll have it by tomorrow," Martha assured him. She'd been Frank's secretary for ten years and had watched him age before her eyes. "Frank?" she buzzed the intercom into his office, "How about a sandwich or something? I'm going out to get a bite when I mail this proposal."

"Nah, don't have time," he grumbled back. "Just a cup of coffee if it's not too much trouble." Frank noticed a burning sensation in his gut as he washed down the last swig of cold, black coffee. In his busyness and concentration he consciously ignored the little flutter and squeezing sensation deep in his chest. He'd been ignoring a lot of things lately, like his wife Susan's gentle suggestions to get a little exercise or to cut back on the caffeine. She just didn't seem to understand all the pressures he had and how much his company depended on him. He was sick and tired of her sweet yet persistent admonishments for him to slow down.

"Frank, darling, I just worry about you," she had whispered to him last Friday night as he lay dozing on the couch with the newspaper in a heap on his lap. "You're just so exhausted at the end of each day. You can't keep up this pace forever!"

Susan hadn't realized how prophetic that statement would be. Martha had returned with Frank's coffee that afternoon only to find him pacing the office clutching his chest. "Ahh, I've got some killer heartburn, Martha. Have any antacids?" he asked as he rubbed his left arm.

"Frank, you don't look good. I'm calling Susan. I think you need to see a doctor!"

"Nah!" he retorted and stopped abruptly, gasping for air as he collapsed in a heap on the floor.

Susan met Frank in the emergency room. His pale, clammy skin frightened her, and she held back tears knowing he would appreciate a strong front. She sent up a silent prayer, "God, I sure hope this will get his attention!"

Frank had become a good example of how our strengths can become our weaknesses. His powerful Choleric personality had always driven him toward success, especially in the business world. Unfortunately, his health had paid the price at the risk of his very life. He was going to have to make a choice. But what would motivate this strong, Choleric man to change? He needed a lifestyle approach that would give him a sense of control, purpose, and accomplishment. Recovering from his mild heart attack gave Frank some time to think about the changes he needed to make.

A few weeks later, Susan came rushing into his room, bright-faced and glowing. Tossing a folded newspaper onto his bed, she quipped, "You need this, Frank. And this time I won't take no for an answer; you are too important to me. Read this and get dressed."

The Melancholy "Method": Karen, Out-of-Shape Graduate Student

Karen sat staring at her computer monitor. She was exhausted. She felt like she'd been working on her thesis for an eternity. This machine had become her constant companion and Friday night date. Her back and neck ached from hunching over her desk for hours on end.

"I've got to get some exercise," she thought. But she knew she wouldn't take the time unless she could really dedicate herself to a complete routine. In her mind, nothing was worth doing unless you did it completely right. So for now her routine was work, study, work, study. At least she would be sure she received the perfect A on this paper.

The sad truth was, once she finished her thesis, her life wouldn't get any more physically active. She had been offered an advanced research position at the university. "Now that's a high-energy job!" she mused. She could imagine herself twenty years from now—a hunched-over, weak, pale old maid.

"Maybe I should get a life," she laughed to herself. The ring of the phone interrupted her thoughts. It was her college friend Elise, inviting her to an old-fashioned picnic complete with three-legged races, volleyball, and croquet. "Okay, okay, Elise," Karen answered, succumbing to her friend's gentle pressure to emerge from her "high-tech" cave. It would be good for her to see sunlight once in a while.

The perfect Melancholy Karen checked one more item off her Saturday morning "to do" list before leaving for the picnic. If she hadn't promised Elise she would show, she would have stayed home and completed every task. She could almost hear her computer audibly calling her from the doorway, "Get back here; you're not done yet!"

She had jumped into all the day's activities with total enthusiasm, figuring she could make up for five years of inactivity in a single afternoon. Her lungs ached as they sucked for more oxygen, not used to this level of demand. She pushed herself to the limit, her competitive spirit pushing her to win at every event. She finally pushed beyond her body's current ability to respond: leaping for the volleyball to make the game point, she heard a loud "pop," and down she went.

"Ouch! No, I can't step on it; I think I've ruptured my Achilles tendon!" Karen had screamed as Elise and two of the stronger guys helped Karen off the field. Recovering from her injury, Karen realized how out of shape she had become. And her nutritional habits were atrocious. She had shelved any healthy habits she had once had and become "tunnel visioned" on getting through school. At twenty-eight, she realized she was more out of shape than some of her active forty-year-old friends.

"Okay, that's it!" she decided. "But where do I start?" She glanced down at the local paper sitting on her desk, and a key word caught her eye. "Hmm, that sounds like me. Maybe I'll check this one out!"

The Phlegmatic "Fallout": Janet, Overweight and Depressed Mother of Three

Janet had grown increasingly frustrated over the years as she struggled to lose weight after the birth of each new baby. Now, at thirty-six with three children, she was at an all-time low both physically and emotionally. The original 10 pounds she added after Nicole, her first child, became 20 after Jonathan, her second. Though she had tried desperately to exercise and diet, she ultimately added another 10 pounds before she was surprised with her last pregnancy. She had felt so hopeless and defeated, she had not even tried to minimize the weight gain during this last pregnancy. When baby Laurel entered the world, Janet was so overweight and depressed, she had a hard time bonding with her.

At her six-week checkup, Janet cringed as the nurse recorded her weight at a whopping 205 pounds. Dr. Kaplan admonished her with a warning when her blood pressure registered at an all-time high. "Janet, it's important to get this under control. Your health is at risk with this kind of blood pressure."

"Dr. Kaplan, I don't know what to do. I've tried every diet out there and failed," she sighed.

"Janet, you have to lose at least 50 pounds. Stop at the reception desk on the way out and I'll have the nurse give you a 1,000-calorie diet. Oh, and you should get some exercise too."

Janet cringed at the thought of another cycle of deprivation and frustration. She'd been down that road many times. A wave of anxiety began to sweep over her just thinking about the enormous task of shedding all this weight. Driving home, she decided that Thursday was not a good day to start this new endeavor. *Monday is always a great day for a new beginning,* she reasoned, eating a last big hamburger with cheese.

As a peaceful Phlegmatic, Janet had always been well liked with a wide variety of friends. Her "go with the flow" personality never ruffled any feathers, and she had sailed through childhood and adolescence with minimal stress. Of course, that is exactly the kind of life a Phlegmatic prefers—smooth, carefree, and peaceful. As a new wife, Janet had discovered that her Melancholy husband, Jim, was more of a challenge than she had realized. His natural desire for perfection and self-discipline gave way to impatience with Janet's expanding waistline and apparent lack of self-control.

She remembered back to the "program" Jim had designed for her to shed her excess weight after their first baby. It was complete with charts and graphs and a detailed menu plan he had sent away for. Janet became easily overwhelmed and gave up after two weeks. Jim had persisted over the next five years, criticizing her adamantly with each new pound. She had withdrawn to the television and sleeping late to avoid Jim's obvious distaste for her enlarging body.

While the kids were at school and Jim was at work, Janet buried her frustration with binge eating. At dinner she would pick at her food and pretend to be dieting. This had become the vicious cycle of her life, and the thought of starting one more futile diet was more than she could bear.

What Janet had not realized through the years was the influence her Phlegmatic personality had on her ability to change lifestyle habits. She had been unsuccessful trying to change using her husband's Melancholy approach. Janet needed a fresh, new approach, one that suited her peaceful nature.

She almost missed the ad as she thumbed through the day's newspaper, but one word caught her attention and she read on.

Sharon, Frank, Karen, and Janet had all read the following newspaper ad:

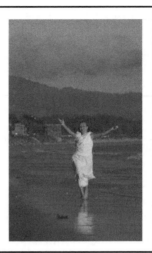
The Workshop

I was excited to greet our workshop guests as I watched the room fill with all sizes, shapes, and ages of people. I could see the looks of anxiety and anticipation on their faces. I was certain many wondered if they were wasting their time looking for another answer to the same old question, "How can I possibly change my habits and body for good?" Janet and her husband found a seat next to Frank and Susan, and they exchanged smiles. Karen had convinced her friend Elise to come along. Sharon and Dan sneaked into the room just as I stepped forward to speak.

"Good evening! My name is Danna and I used to be a compulsive-eating couch potato weighing about 25 pounds more than I do tonight." A few people chuckled as I continued, "Is there anyone here who would like to change at least one little thing about their body or habits?" Hands went up all over the room, along with snickers and laughs. "So I guess we have something in common," I added.

"In a group this size, there will be many who want to lose weight, increase their fitness, or improve energy levels. Let's face it, our body is our vehicle for life. If it doesn't look or run well, life cannot be lived to its fullest. I'm sure most of you have owned more than one car in your life. Unfortunately, this body is the only one you'll ever have this side of heaven. You can't trade it in. You wouldn't be here tonight if you had fully figured out how to maintain a healthy, high-energy body. So what do you think the problem is? Why is it so hard to change habits? I propose to you that much of the problem in living healthfully lies in your approach.

"Each of you came to this lecture because you saw an advertisement in the local newspaper. What was it that drew you here? First, you had a need to make a change in your lifestyle or habits for one reason or another. Second, a word or phrase probably caught your attention. Do the words *fun*, *perfect*, *control*, or *peace* speak to any of you?" I could see finger pokes, elbow jabs, and raised eyebrows around the room.

"These words each describe one of the primary motivators peculiar to each of four personality types." After a brief overview of the four personalities, I explained how focusing on our unique personality could dramatically impact our ability to make effective lifestyle changes.

Each person was tested to determine his or her primary personality. Then the group was divided by personality into four smaller segments. Each person was coached to develop their own customized lifestyle plan based on their goals and personality type.

Everyone was encouraged to support one another in their differences. I told them, "An understanding of your unique personalities will help you better accept why your wife, husband, or friend can't do things just like you do. Accept and celebrate the differences, and we can all reach our goals with a whole lot less heartache and frustration!

"Remember, we have to base all lifestyle change on some fundamental truths about the human body," I cautioned them. "You need to have a healthy, long-term approach. Ask yourself the question, 'Can I live with this behavior for the rest of my life? Would it be healthful, practical, or even possible?' If the answer is no, don't add it to your plan! If you are unsure about what healthy eating and exercising look like, get educated *before* designing your plan. Then use the Personality-Powered Lifestyle Guide to help you create an action plan that works for your unique temperament."

Solutions

Sanguine Sharon was so excited she couldn't wait to get started. She began enthusiastically sharing her new ideas and plan with her husband, Dan, and caught herself in mid-sentence. "Hmmm," she pondered out loud, "here I go again, taking off on a new program without measuring the cost. I think the first thing I'll do is get an accountability partner and take one step at a time." She was encouraged that she could make healthy changes by taking small, consistent steps. She understood she didn't have to compromise her long-term health or budget in the process.

Choleric Frank had been a little impatient with the introductions and leery of the new "diet and exercise plan" he was sure would be prescribed for him before the evening was over. He had to admit he was relieved and very pleased he would be encouraged to develop and implement his own plan. After all, he did like to be in control. He didn't miss the gentle stare from his wife when I reminded the Cholerics not to jump into their new lifestyle changes with too much vigor. He knew from his professional experience how that had been his undoing. This time he would take some of his energy and channel it slowly into this new lifestyle approach.

Melancholy Karen had already begun a list of things she would do this week to find the best workout equipment or gyms in the area. She had even created a "healthy" shopping list when she was stopped by a special caution to all the Melancholy personalities. I warned, "You Melancholy's may take all this so seriously that you'll spend more time planning and researching your new lifestyle than actually doing it. Everything doesn't have to be perfect before you start. Enjoy the journey of developing your new habits and fine-tune it as you go. However, you will enjoy and get great satisfaction from keeping accurate charts of your activities and progress. Go for it!"

Phlegmatic Janet was relieved to know she didn't have to go on another restrictive diet to lose her excess weight. She understood that she would always do better with a simple "one step at a time" approach. She also recognized the need for a partner or personal trainer other than her perfect Melancholy husband, Jim. She needed someone who could keep her accountable to those day-by-day baby steps without exerting too much pressure. Jim also gained some insights and made a promise to himself and to Janet not to try to make her do things "his way." That alone gave her tremendous comfort and encouragement.

What's Your Personality Type?

The following pages include a personality profile and scoring sheet to determine your unique personality type. Typically, you are a combination of styles, with one or two being more dominant. Be as honest as you can, and if you're not sure which word best describes you, ask your spouse or a good friend who knows you well. Have fun with this!

Personality Profile

Directions—In each of the following rows of *four words across*, place an X in front of the *one* word that most often applies to you. Continue through all forty lines; be sure each number is marked. If you are not sure which word "most applies," ask a spouse or a friend, and think of what your answer would have been *when you were a child*.

Strengths

1 ___ Adventurous	___ Adaptable	___ Animated	___ Analytical
2 ___ Persistent	___ Playful	___ Persuasive	___ Peaceful
3 ___ Submissive	___ Self-sacrificing	___ Sociable	___ Strong-willed
4 ___ Considerate	___ Controlled	___ Competitive	___ Convincing
5 ___ Refreshing	___ Respectful	___ Reserved	___ Resourceful
6 ___ Satisfied	___ Sensitive	___ Self-reliant	___ Spirited
7 ___ Planner	___ Patient	___ Positive	___ Promoter
8 ___ Sure	___ Spontaneous	___ Scheduled	___ Shy
9 ___ Orderly	___ Obliging	___ Outspoken	___ Optimistic
10 ___ Friendly	___ Faithful	___ Funny	___ Forceful
11 ___ Daring	___ Delightful	___ Diplomatic	___ Detailed

12 ___ Cheerful	___ Consistent	___ Cultured	___ Confident
13 ___ Idealistic	___ Independent	___ Inoffensive	___ Inspiring
14 ___ Demonstrative	___ Decisive	___ Dry humor	___ Deep
15 ___ Mediator	___ Musical	___ Mover	___ Mixes easily
16 ___ Thoughtful	___ Tenacious	___ Talker	___ Tolerant
17 ___ Listener	___ Loyal	___ Leader	___ Lively
18 ___ Contented	___ Chief	___ Chartmaker	___ Cute
19 ___ Perfectionist	___ Pleasant	___ Productive	___ Popular
20 ___ Bouncy	___ Bold	___ Behaved	___ Balanced

Weaknesses

21 ___ Blank	___ Bashful	___ Brassy	___ Bossy
22 ___ Undisciplined	___ Unsympathetic	___ Unenthusiastic	___ Unforgiving
23 ___ Reticent	___ Resentful	___ Resistant	___ Repetitious
24 ___ Fussy	___ Fearful	___ Forgetful	___ Frank
25 ___ Impatient	___ Insecure	___ Indecisive	___ Interrupts
26 ___ Unpopular	___ Uninvolved	___ Unpredictable	___ Unaffectionate
27 ___ Headstrong	___ Haphazard	___ Hard to please	___ Hesitant
28 ___ Plain	___ Pessimistic	___ Proud	___ Permissive
29 ___ Angered easily	___ Aimless	___ Argumentative	___ Alienated
30 ___ Naive	___ Negative attitude	___ Nervy	___ Nonchalant
31 ___ Worrier	___ Withdrawn	___ Workaholic	___ Wants credit
32 ___ Too sensitive	___ Tactless	___ Timid	___ Talkative
33 ___ Doubtful	___ Disorganized	___ Domineering	___ Depressed
34 ___ Inconsistent	___ Introvert	___ Intolerant	___ Indifferent
35 ___ Messy	___ Moody	___ Mumbles	___ Manipulative
36 ___ Slow	___ Stubborn	___ Show-off	___ Skeptical
37 ___ Loner	___ Lord over others	___ Lazy	___ Loud

38 ___ Sluggish	___ Suspicious	___ Short-tempered	___ Scatterbrained
39 ___ Revengeful	___ Restless	___ Reluctant	___ Rash
40 ___ Compromising	___ Critical	___ Crafty	___ Changeable

Personality Scoring Sheet

Now transfer all your X's to the corresponding words on the Personality Scoring Sheet and add up your totals. For example, if you checked Animated on the profile, check it on the scoring sheet. (Note: The words are in a different order on the profile and the scoring sheet.)

Strengths

Popular Sanguine	Powerful Choleric	Perfect Melancholy	Peaceful Phlegmatic
1 ___ Animated	___ Adventurous	___ Analytical	___ Adaptable
2 ___ Playful	___ Persuasive	___ Persistent	___ Peaceful
3 ___ Sociable	___ Strong-willed	___ Self-sacrificing	___ Submissive
4 ___ Convincing	___ Competitive	___ Considerate	___ Controlled
5 ___ Refreshing	___ Resourceful	___ Respectful	___ Reserved
6 ___ Spirited	___ Self-reliant	___ Sensitive	___ Satisfied
7 ___ Promoter	___ Positive	___ Planner	___ Patient
8 ___ Spontaneous	___ Sure	___ Scheduled	___ Shy
9 ___ Optimistic	___ Outspoken	___ Orderly	___ Obliging
10 ___ Funny	___ Forceful	___ Faithful	___ Friendly
11 ___ Delightful	___ Daring	___ Detailed	___ Diplomatic
12 ___ Cheerful	___ Confident	___ Cultured	___ Consistent
13 ___ Inspiring	___ Independent	___ Idealistic	___ Inoffensive
14 ___ Demonstrative	___ Decisive	___ Deep	___ Dry humor
15 ___ Mixes easily	___ Mover	___ Musical	___ Mediator

16 ___ Talker	___ Tenacious	___ Thoughtful	___ Tolerant
17 ___ Lively	___ Leader	___ Loyal	___ Listener
18 ___ Cute	___ Chief	___ Chartmaker	___ Contented
19 ___ Popular	___ Productive	___ Perfectionist	___ Pleasant
20 ___ Bouncy	___ Bold	___ Behaved	___ Balanced

Totals—Strengths

___   ___   ___   ___

Weaknesses

Popular Sanguine	Powerful Choleric	Perfect Melancholy	Peaceful Phlegmatic
21 ___ Brassy	___ Bossy	___ Bashful	___ Blank
22 ___ Undisciplined	___ Unsympathetic	___ Unforgiving	___ Unenthusiastic
23 ___ Repetitious	___ Resistant	___ Resentful	___ Reticent
24 ___ Forgetful	___ Frank	___ Fussy	___ Fearful
25 ___ Interrupts	___ Impatient	___ Insecure	___ Indecisive
26 ___ Unpredictable	___ Unaffectionate	___ Unpopular	___ Uninvolved
27 ___ Haphazard	___ Headstrong	___ Hard to please	___ Hesitant
28 ___ Permissive	___ Proud	___ Pessimistic	___ Plain
29 ___ Angered easily	___ Argumentative	___ Alienated	___ Aimless
30 ___ Naive	___ Nervy	___ Negative attitude	___ Nonchalant
31 ___ Wants credit	___ Workaholic	___ Withdrawn	___ Worrier
32 ___ Talkative	___ Tactless	___ Too sensitive	___ Timid
33 ___ Disorganized	___ Domineering	___ Depressed	___ Doubtful
34 ___ Inconsistent	___ Intolerant	___ Introvert	___ Indifferent
35 ___ Messy	___ Manipulative	___ Moody	___ Mumbles
36 ___ Show-off	___ Stubborn	___ Skeptical	___ Slow
37 ___ Loud	___ Lord over others	___ Loner	___ Lazy

38 ___ Scatterbrained ___ Short-tempered   ___ Suspicious   ___ Sluggish

39 ___ Restless   ___ Rash   ___ Revengeful   ___ Reluctant

40 ___ Changeable   ___ Crafty   ___ Critical   ___ Compromising

Totals—Weaknesses

___   ___   ___   ___

Combined Totals

___   ___   ___   ___

Lifestyle Guides for the Four Personalities

The Popular Sanguine . . . Just Wants to Have Fun!

Do:

- Gain a fundamental base of knowledge about nutrition and exercise
- Choose a fun book or fast-paced program and get started
- Find an accountability partner to help keep you on track

Don't:

- Go on a diet!
- Try quick-fix, short-term solutions
- Buy every new piece of exercise equipment

Exercise:

- Find a variety of activities you enjoy
- Turn exercise into a social event—like walks with friends or an aerobics class
- Schedule time to exercise each week and stick to it
- Give yourself lots of variety
- Enjoy the positive feedback from wearing your Caltrac

Nutrition:

- Follow the energy formula: breakfast, water, fiber, protein, and limited caffeine and sugar intake
- Keep it simple with a solid nutritional base
- Find creative ways to cut calories that you can live with
- Plan for "fun foods" and stick with your plan

Stress:

- Avoid over-commitment; learn to have realistic expectations
- Slow down and purposely relax
- Enjoy some time alone

Motivation:

- "Be transformed by the renewing of your mind" (Rom. 12:2)
- Specifically visualize your goals, write them down, and read them daily
- Ask for feedback from your accountability partner
- Turn off any negative "self-talk"
- Use positive self-talk tapes

The Powerful Choleric . . . Just Wants to Have Control!

Do:

- Gain a fundamental base of knowledge about nutrition and exercise
- Be patient with yourself and your progress
- Give yourself adequate time for results

Don't:

- Go on a diet!
- Have unrealistic expectations

- Go overboard with exercise; balance is the key
- Forget to warm up and stretch to prevent injuries

Exercise:

- Choose simple and effective exercises that are time efficient
- Create a realistic exercise schedule and alternate activities for best results
- Early morning exercise may be best (you only have to shower once)
- Find a class, trainer, or coach that will provide the challenge you need

Nutrition:

- Follow the energy formula: breakfast, water, fiber, protein, and limited caffeine and sugar intake
- Make some simple, basic changes in your overall nutrition to meet your goals
- Eat breakfast every day—no matter how busy you are
- Stop eating lunch while you work and enjoy your meals
- Avoid heavy, late-evening dinners

Stress:

- Slow down and take time to experience the "small stuff"
- Schedule "down time" into your life
- Use proactive stress-busters like walks, journaling, massage, and fun!
- Get adequate sleep and avoid caffeine

Motivation:

- "Be transformed by the renewing of your mind" (Rom. 12:2)
- Determine your physical objectives and weigh the cost

- Create a realistic action plan and schedule it into your life
- Use positive self-talk tapes
- Your greatest motivation will be results, so . . . just do it!

The Perfect Melancholy . . . Just Wants to Have Perfection!

Do:

- Gain a fundamental base of knowledge about nutrition and exercise
- Find a comprehensive, detailed program or book as a resource
- Begin taking action *before* you have all the answers
- Schedule your new lifestyle changes into your calendar
- Take a break now and then
- Accept that others may choose to do things differently

Don't:

- Go on a diet!
- Expect perfection or procrastinate until you have the perfect solution
- Go overboard with your new lifestyle
- Expect others to readily participate in your "new program"

Exercise:

- Use your Caltrac and log your progress
- Choose a variety of activities
- Select a club or gym that offers a comprehensive orientation
- Consider a personal trainer to fine-tune your fitness

Nutrition:

- Follow the energy formula: breakfast, water, fiber, protein, and limited caffeine and sugar intake

- Start with the basics and modify your diet as you learn the facts
- Use your organizational skills to create healthful meal plans and shopping lists
- Keep a log of your new habits and chart daily
- Relax your standards occasionally to enjoy life's little pleasures

Stress:

- Give yourself permission to be human
- Realize life is not an all or nothing venture—little things count
- Practice "letting go" of perfection and feeling okay

Motivation:

- "Be transformed by the renewing of your mind" (Rom. 12:2)
- Examine your beliefs and learn to let go of the lies
- Celebrate small victories and keep records of your small steps
- Listen to healthy self-talk audio tapes

The Peaceful Phlegmatic . . . Just Wants to Have Peace

Do:

- Gain a fundamental base of knowledge about nutrition and exercise
- Find a class or book that will instruct you step by step
- Take one step at a time . . . it's okay
- Keep your plans simple
- Take small steps each and every day

Don't:

- Go on a diet!
- Wait until Monday or the first of the month to begin your new habits

- Get overwhelmed with too many details
- Become apathetic about your health

Exercise:

- Find a workout partner or trainer to keep you accountable
- Make appointments with yourself to work out, and keep them
- Maintain your own pace and don't succumb to others' pressures or programs
- Find creative ways to move more each day—you don't have to sweat!

Nutrition:

- Follow the energy formula: breakfast, water, fiber, protein, and limited caffeine and sugar intake
- Watch out for grazing with sedentary activities like TV
- Choose one or two dietary changes at a time
- Shop with a list and a plan
- Think about what you are going to eat beforehand

Motivation:

- "Be transformed by the renewing of your mind" (Rom. 12:2)
- Ask your workout partner or trainer to help you evaluate your progress
- Celebrate even small successes
- Believe in your ability to "stick with it"
- Listen to "healthy self-talk" audio tapes at least twice each day
- Remember, "Garbage in . . . garbage out. Good stuff in . . . good stuff out!"

Optional Section:
Logging for Success

In This Section:

Why Take Time to Log?

Statistics show that people who log their progress daily are the most successful. Take a few minutes each day to record your food choices, activity, and workouts. Seeing your own triumphs in writing will inspire and motivate you. It's documented proof of all your hard work!

The *Scale Down* Daily Success Plan

I have included a copy of the *Scale Down* Daily Success Plan. The log will give you tremendous insight into your own habits. We all say, "I should eat less," but do you really know how much you're eating now? We all say, "I should exercise more," but do you have any idea how many calories you're currently burning each day? Your log will help you pinpoint exactly where your problem areas are and help you set concrete, achievable goals.

To help you get a realistic picture of exactly what you're eating and how much you're moving, you may want to keep a daily log as you go through the program. Whether you're eating too much fat, eating too many calories, skimping on fiber, or neglecting to exercise, your log will help you see a snapshot of your habits and help you hold yourself accountable to new behaviors. Focus on the changes in your habits, not what the scale says or the size of your muscles. Your body will always respond to *consistent* action. As I've said before, do the right things long enough and your best body will follow.

SCALE DOWN DAILY SUCCESS PLAN

DATE	TODAY'S NUTRITION GOALS	*Cals*	*Carbo*	*Pro*	*Fat*	*Fiber* 30 grams	*MultiVitamins* ❑ 1st ❑ 2nd *Antioxidant* ❑ Yes ❑ No		
MEALS	**FOOD ITEMS**	**Cals**	**Carbo**	**Pro**	**Fat**	**Fiber**	**Hunger Before** (Rate 1-5)	**Hunger After** (Rate 1-5)	**WATER**
Breakfast									❑
									❑
SNACK									❑
Lunch									❑
									❑
									❑
SNACK									❑
Dinner									❑
									❑
									❑
									❑
SNACK									❑
TOTALS	# Fruits _____ # Vegies _____								

ACTIVITIES – Describe what you did today in these lifestyle areas

SPIRITUAL	
MENTAL	Listened to SELF TALK: ❑ ❑ ❑ ❑
PHYSICAL	❑ AEROBIC How long? ❑ MUSCLE WORK Describe: ❑ STRETCHING
ENERGY	❑ Great! ❑ Good ❑ Fair ❑ Poor
SLEEP	# of hours lastnight: _____ Rested today: ❑ Yes ❑ No
CALTRAC LOG	Cals IN / Cals OUT / Active/ACTM Cals / NET / Cumulative (+-)

What went well? _____

Ways to improve tomorrow: _____

Optional Section:
Caltrac, Your Personal Activity Coach

In This Section:

Monitors, Pedometers, and Other Tools

Caltrac: Getting Acquainted

Action Plan for Losing One Pound of Fat per Week

Logging Your Daily Progress

Monitors, Pedometers, and Other Tools

There are a wide variety of tools on the market that may be helpful in moving you toward a healthier, more active lifestyle. Heart rate monitors help you get a safe aerobic workout and stay in your specific target heart rate zone. Pedometers measure how many steps you take and can motivate you toward more movement. Many treadmills, stationary bikes, and other cardio equipment offer a "calorie burn" monitor built into the equipment's computer. These can be helpful to give you a general idea of how many calories you are burning but are quite inaccurate unless you are able to input your specific information such as age, weight, height, and sex.

After years of evaluation, I have found the Caltrac to be the most comprehensive and accurate tool available. That is not to say it is the only tool or that the others have no benefit. It can be used in almost all activities (except for water sports). Because I have had thousands of clients sing its praises as a highly useful tool, I have chosen to include this special section for those who are using the Caltrac. Though the Caltrac comes with a good user manual and helpful video, the information in this section is very specific and in response to over a decade of using this tool.

Caltrac: Getting Acquainted

If you have chosen to use a Caltrac activity monitor, it's time to get acquainted with it. If you're considering one, this information will be helpful to you as well. Caltrac is a mini-computer that converts motion into calorie burn with 97 to 99 percent accuracy for most activities. The accelerometer that picks up all your movement is the same technology used in jet engines to sense even the slightest motion change.

The Caltrac interprets your activity and translates it very accurately into calorie burn based on your personal statistics—that is, your age, height, weight, and sex. Caltrac has been used extensively in universities across the United States to measure the activity levels of people of all ages. Nothing else like it is on the market.

In addition to calculating all your motion into calorie burn, Caltrac is also constantly adding in your non-movement calories (or resting metabolic rate). The Caltrac will update your calorie burn information every two minutes. If your information hasn't changed, you haven't completed a full two-minute cycle. You will be able to see just how much you moved and the total number of calories you burned each day. It is an excellent personal coach and reality checker. You may be surprised how much or how little you burn. But your body knows *exactly* what you're burning and exactly how many calories you're eating.

The best way to use the Caltrac is to take one week at a time and become familiar with using it and logging your results. You will be amazed how motivating it is to watch your activity calories increase.

We are very much like little children who get stars on their progress charts for good behavior. Caltrac will help you develop a new attitude about moving. Every time you move your body mass through space, you burn calories. Park a little farther from the grocery store. Walk to the post office or take your dog for one more lap around the block. You'll be amazed how little changes in behavior can add up in a big way over time.

Please note: Caltrac is very sturdy and resilient. However, do not wear your Caltrac in water (or accidentally drop it in the toilet). It is *not* necessary to wear it to bed. The few calories you miss from tossing and turning are not worth the discomfort of rolling over on the little contraption.

Understanding Caltrac Function Modes

Cals Used: This is the total number of calories you have burned for the day and includes your resting and activity calories.

Cals: This is the number of calories you have eaten. (Please note: You must tell the Caltrac what you've eaten by entering your calories throughout the day or at the end of the day if you want to use this feature.)

Net Cals: The reality hits here! If you enter the calories you eat, then Caltrac does the math for you. You will see if you are ahead or behind in the count. If you've eaten more than you've burned, the excess is stored as fat. You don't want that!

ACTM: This mode simply allows you to visualize how the Caltrac senses motion and translates it to calorie burn. As you shake your Caltrac, you can see the number increase very quickly. When shaken aggressively, the ACTM number should easily increase to three hundred or more. This demonstrates that the motion sensor is working correctly.

ACTM Cals Used: This is the number of calories you have burned *from activity*. It's also the one you have control over. The more you move, the higher the number will go over the day. You'll stay on track best if you aim for a minimum activity calorie burn each day.

Using Pedal and Power Modes

Caltrac interprets your motion or activity into calories. For activities when your hips are essentially stationary, like riding a bike or lifting weights, it needs to be put on the appropriate mode to more accurately interpret and measure your calorie burn.

PEDAL MODE

This mode is accessed by pressing the "bicycle button" and shows it is on by the "PM" on the display. When on, it is essentially calculating your calories about three times higher than in the regular mode to more accurately interpret the following types of activities:

- [ ] Bike
- [ ] Rowing machine
- [ ] Treadmill at 12 percent grade or higher
- [ ] NordicTrack
- [ ] StairMaster

POWER MODE

This mode is accessed by pressing the "dumbbell button" and shows it is on by the flashing "PM" on the display. When on, it is essentially calculating your calories two times higher than in the regular mode to more accurately interpret the following types of activities:

- [ ] Heavy muscle work
- [ ] Weight lifting
- [ ] Heavy gardening
- [ ] Treadmill at 6 to 11 percent grade

Very important note: Remember to put the Caltrac back on regular mode after stopping the special activity. You do this by hitting the bicycle or weight button again. Failure to do so will give you an inaccurate calorie reading for the day.

Using Caltrac: Week One

In week one, you should get some important baseline data. Try to simulate an average week in terms of activity. If you have been sedentary for a long time, this is not the week to increase your activity. You want to get a realistic picture of your average calorie burn so you can give yourself a new "energy prescription" next week. That will be the time to start "putting on the burn."

Wear your Caltrac daily on your waistband or belt. This week, begin logging your calorie burn using the chart on page 155 and focus on three things:

☐ Determine your active calorie burn, which is displayed as "CALS USED ACTM" on your Caltrac monitor.

☐ Note your total burn (activity and resting calories) at the end of the day. This is displayed as "CALS USED" on your Caltrac.

☐ Every day, record how many ACTM (active) calories you have burned as well as your total CALS USED. Then zero out your Caltrac and start another 24-hour cycle.

Using Caltrac: Week Two

Evaluate yourself after your first week wearing the Caltrac. Did any of the information surprise you? Many people don't realize how few calories they burn from activity. Larger individuals, especially men, will burn many more calories than smaller individuals. As your body weight decreases, so will the calories you burn in all activities. The Caltrac will be most beneficial to you as a tool to objectively measure your increase in activity.

DETERMINE YOUR RMR USING CALTRAC

Now it's time to learn a little more about your calorie-burning body by determining your resting metabolic rate (RMR). That is the number of calories you burn each 24 hours simply doing nothing. This is the number of calories your body needs every day just to survive. It is also the minimum number of calories you should eat each day to avoid damaging your metabolism.

FIVE EASY STEPS

1. Zero out your Caltrac.
2. Place it on your bedside table for 8 hours.
3. After 8 hours, write down the number on the "Cals Used" display and enter it below by the (a).
4. Then multiply (a) by 3 and enter that number below by the (b).

   (a) _____ x 3 = _____ (b)

5. Now multiply (b) by 0.9 to get your RMR:

   (b) _____ x 0.9 = _____ (your RMR)

GOING FOR THE BURN

Once you have established your true calorie burn average, begin to notch up your activity. Set a goal to increase your average activity by at least 100 calories per day. If you're up to a real challenge, I encourage you to go as high as 200. This will be harder if you are a petite woman and relatively easy if you are a 200-pound man. So set your objectives accordingly. Find out how long it takes you to burn that extra 100 calories. Is it ten minutes, fifteen, or even twenty? What kind of activities do you enjoy? Where do you burn the most calories? Have fun. Try something new.

Many people think that you have to go to the gym or get all sweaty to burn calories. It just isn't true. While we gain obvious benefits from strengthening our cardiovascular system or toning up our muscles, even moderate, non-exercise activity burns calories.

Just imagine farmers at the turn of the twentieth century. How many stopped in the middle of the field to check whether their heart rate was in their "target zone"? Getting our heart rate into a target zone for fifteen to twenty minutes three times a week is only necessary because the rest of our day is so sedentary. Cumulative moderate activity can have a very beneficial effect if we get enough activity. By wearing the Caltrac, you will see that no activity is wasted.

You have to decide on both your fitness and weight management goals. If you want to be a more efficient calorie burner, you'll want to improve your fitness level. Then you can move at a higher intensity and burn calories more efficiently. Walking a mile or running a mile burns about the same number of calories. The runner just gets finished faster!

Let's Review

1. Calculate your resting metabolic rate to determine the minimum number of calories you should eat every day.
2. Never eat less than your RMR.
3. Determine your daily averages for ACTM and CALS USED calories.
4. Begin to notch up your ACTM calorie burn by 100, 200, or even 300 calories per day.
5. Create a list of activities you will do this week and answer the following questions to help you create an action plan:
   a. What activity are you willing to do for ten minutes each morning? _____
   b. Where could you walk this week instead of drive?

   _____
   c. Will you park farther away?

   _____
   d. How about a walking visit with a friend instead of coffee or lunch? _____
   e. Will you exercise or stretch while you watch television?

   _____
   f. How many elevators or escalators could you avoid this week?

   _____
   g. What other ideas do you have?

   _____
6. Continue to log your ACTM and CALS USED each night.

The Ultimate "Reality Check"

If you are up to the challenge and have a personality that likes to track details, then you can use the Caltrac to its fullest capacity. To do so, you need to track not only how many calories you are burning each day but also how many you are eating. I understand that this exercise is not for everyone. It is also not a true "lifestyle" approach. Instead, it is what I call a "reality check." By tracking exactly what you are eating and burning, you can quickly identify when you are off track and take action to eat less or move more to bring yourself into balance.

I recommend this type of lifestyle modification if you are up to the initial challenge of learning how to become an excellent calorie counter and really want to get to the root of your calorie burn challenges.

Action Plan for Losing One Pound of Fat per Week

1. **Eat the number of calories representing your resting metabolic rate (up to 2,000 calories per day).** It is important to include a wide variety of healthy choices and keep your fat intake to 20–25 percent of your total calories. (For 1,500 calories, that would be about 33 grams of fat per day.)
2. **Move at least 500 activity (ACTM) calories per day.** If you move more than that, you can eat more or lose more than one pound per week.
3. **Enter the calories you eat into your Caltrac.** Note your NET CALS number throughout the day. What is your NET CALS goal (in vs. out) for the end of the day? 500 net calories per day x 7 days = 3,500 calories per week or one pound of fat. However, in order to support your metabolism, you must have ACTM (activity) calories or exceed your NET calories. For example, if your NET CALS at the end of the day are 600, then your ACTM calories should be at least 600. Otherwise, you will be eating too few calories to support a healthy metabolism over the long haul.
4. **Look at the big picture.** Don't micromanage your activity or your eating. You can have several days of negative NET CALS and still

burn off a pound of fat by making up the difference on other days. Don't sabotage yourself by expecting perfection. (See my example on the next page.)

5. **Set realistic goals** and find an accountability partner.

6. **Don't give up!** Changing your behavior takes time. Just try to do a little better tomorrow. Three steps forward and two steps back means you are still moving in a positive direction.

Use your Caltrac as a personal "accountability" coach. It will give you an honest reality check so that you can keep focused on the truth. Enjoy becoming a more active person. Soon you will be a leaner, healthier person also!

Logging Your Daily Progress

On the next page, you'll see an example of one month when I wore the Caltrac every day and logged my activity. If you look at the chart, you'll see that even though the average daily net calorie difference was only 113, I still burned almost 1 pound of body fat (3,500 calories) in one month.

CALTRAC LOG EXAMPLE

Taken from 1 month recording by Danna Demetre, RN

DAY	CALS IN	CALS USED	ACTIVE ACTM CALS	NET CALS	CUM. +/−
1	1866	1875	361	9	9
2	1842	1844	396	2	11
3	2121	2244	750	123	134
4	2300	1800	360	−500	−366
5	2133	2186	746	53	−313
6	1975	2000	550	25	−288
7	1952	2327	688	375	87
8	1926	1989	549	63	150
9	1943	1946	456	3	153
10	1940	1950	460	10	163
11	2026	1851	547	−175	−12
12	1943	1946	456	3	−9
13	1817	1834	263	17	8
14	2403	2294	802	−109	−101
15	1725	1860	347	135	34
16	1686	2208	559	522	556
17	1728	1820	334	92	648
18	1850	1910	390	60	708
19	2100	2485	1001	385	1093
20	1946	1980	481	34	1127
21	1842	2197	692	355	1482
22	1746	1842	287	96	1578
23	1498	2045	547	547	2125
24	2005	2105	601	100	2225
25	1750	1940	502	190	2415
26	1950	2220	780	270	2685
27	2000	2100	600	100	2785
28	1850	1950	410	100	2885
29	1578	1862	422	284	3169
30	1625	1835	394	210	3379
31					
TOTALS	57066	60445	15731	3379	3379
AVERAGE	1902	2015	524	113	113

CALTRAC DAILY LOG

Month _____   Goal _____

DAY	CALS IN	CALS USED	ACTIVE ACTM CALS	NET CALS	CUM. +/−
1					
2					
3					
4					
5					
6					
7					
8					
9					
10					
11					
12					
13					
14					
15					
16					
17					
18					
19					
20					
21					
22					
23					
24					
25					
26					
27					
28					
29					
30					
31					
TOTALS					
AVERAGE					

Danna's encouraging message *is now available in* a curriculum for small groups!

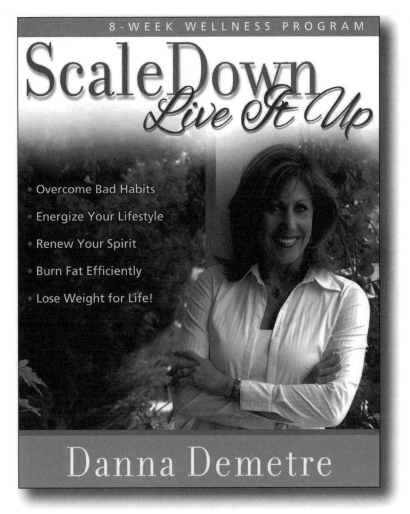

The *Scale Down—Live It Up* curriculum includes:

- a revised and updated edition of the best-selling *Scale Down*
- a DVD featuring six live sessions of Danna Demetre's wellness seminar
- the eight-week *Scale Down—Live It Up Wellness Workbook*
- a 48-page leader's guide